Musicians
Prevention of

A SINGULAR AUDIOLOGY TEXT

Jeffery L. Danhauer, Ph.D.
Audiology Editor

Musicians and the Prevention of Hearing Loss

Marshall Chasin, M.Sc., Aud(C), FAAA
Audiologist

Director of Auditory Research
Centre for Human Performance and Health Promotion
Hamilton, Ontario, Canada

Co-ordinator of Research
Canadian Hearing Society
Toronto, Ontario, Canada

Instructor in the Department of Linguistics
University of Toronto
Toronto, Ontario, Canada

Honourary Lecturer
Department of Communicative Disorders
University of Western Ontario
London, Ontario, Canada

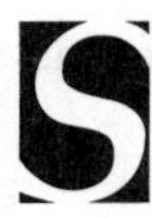

SINGULAR PUBLISHING GROUP, INC.
SAN DIEGO · LONDON

Singular Publishing Group, Inc.
4284 41st Street
San Diego, California 92105-1197

19 Compton Terrace
London, N1 2UN, UK

Typeset in 10/12 Palatino by So Cal Graphics
Printed in the United States of America by McNaughton & Gunn

Library of Congress Cataloging-in-Publication Data

Chasin, Marshall.
Musicians and the prevention of hearing loss / Marshall Chasin.
p. cm.
Includes bibliographical references and index.
ISBN 1-56593-626-4
1. Deafness, Noise induced—Prevention. 2. Musicians—Wounds and injuries—Prevention. I. Title.
RF293.5.C46 1996 96–1122
617.8'008'878—dc20 CIP

Contents

Preface		vii
Chapter 1	Hearing and Hearing Loss—An Introduction	1
Chapter 2	Factors Affecting Hearing Loss	25
Chapter 3	Development of Acoustic Principles	43
Chapter 4	The Physics of Musical Instruments	61
Chapter 5	Hearing Protection	83
Chapter 6	Clinical Assessment of Musicians—Audiologist as a Detective	103
Chapter 7	Room Acoustics	121
Chapter 8	Clinical and Environmental Strategies to Reduce Music Exposure	133
Chapter 9	The Human Performance Approach to Prevention	149
Appendix I	Clinical Information	157
Appendix II	Resources and Service Development	167
References		171
Index		181

Preface

An underlying postulate of this book is that almost any musical environment can be made safe, yet musically acceptable. A combination of ear protection, monitoring devices, and environmental strategies are accepted by a wide range of musicians.

Musicians and the Prevention of Hearing Loss is an axiomatically consistent book that is not full of mathematical formulae. Indeed there are only four in the entire book and these are merely to be viewed as summarizing tools for those factors that affect a specific acoustic behaviour. No prior knowledge of mathematics nor acoustics is required. This book is therefore as readable by a musician as it is by an audiologist or a sound engineer. A unique feature of this book is the wide use of case examples and music spectra from a range of musicians and instruments.

There are nine chapters and two appendixes in the book. Chapter 1 is an introduction to hearing and hearing loss that covers a range of topics of special interest to the counseling of musicians. Chapter 2 is a critical analysis of the relevant research pertaining to factors that can affect hearing. Chapter 3 covers the development of those acoustic principles found in the study of musical instruments, ear protection, and the performing environment. Chapter 4 covers the physics of musical instruments with a focus on those aspects important for the assessment of the musician. Chapter 5 covers the development and assessment of ear protection for those in the performing arts. Chapter 6 is a clinical approach to the assessment of musicians, with case studies. Chapter 7 discusses the science of room acoustics and appropriate modifications. Chapter 8 overviews clinical and environmental strategies that can be implemented to reduce the potential of hearing loss among musicians, yet still allow the environment to be musically acceptable. Chapter 9 discusses many of the issues surrounding the general approach to musicians and the need for individual assessments in most cases. The two appendixes cover information important for the clinical assessment (Appendix I) and service development in the performing arts industry (Appendix II).

Chapter 7 has been co-written with Bill Gastmeier, who is an acoustical engineer. Bill has done extensive work in the modification of performance halls for the performing arts. Dr. John Chong contributed the final chapter on the human performance approach to prevention. John is the medical director of the Centre for Human Performance and Health Promotion (also known as the musicians' clinic) and, other than being a good friend, has taught me much about music.

I would also like to acknowledge Elliott Berger, Bill Cole, Mead Killion, James Hall III, and my editor Jeffery Danhauer, for their discussions and comments on this text. A thank-you also goes to Thong Ling for his artistic abilities.

Special thanks go to my wife, Joanne, and children, Courtney, Meredith, and Shaun for their support and putting up with a "preoccupied" husband and father during the writing of this book.

A portion of the royalties from the sale of this book will go to support the Foundation for Health in the Arts to be used for the education of musicians and the prevention of performing arts injuries.

Dedication

In memory of my friend and colleague
Harold Janzen, M.Sc. (1956–1995)

CHAPTER
1

Hearing and Hearing Loss—An Introduction

INTRODUCTION

Depending on one's perspective, musicians are either a psychophysicist's dream or an audiologist's greatest nightmare. Clinical work with musicians incorporates the study of psychophysical characteristics, which are typically only read about in scholarly journals. Subject areas such as distortion, equal loudness contours, loudness summation, and tinnitus are routine topics in the assessment and the counseling of musicians.

The purpose of this introductory chapter is to provide a basis for the nomenclature, some definitions, and an anatomical model—all of which will be used as a framework in subsequent chapters. This chapter is not intended to provide an in-depth analysis of the physics and psychophysics of music; rather it addresses the salient features and phenomena in a non-mathematical but consistent manner. A physiological basis is provided to answer many of the typical questions a musician may pose. Three psychophysical phenomena are especially important for the education of the musician: equal loudness contours, loudness summation, and diplacusis.

SOUND AND ITS ANALYSIS

In order to understand hearing, several characteristics of sound and its analysis need to be reviewed. *Sound* can be thought of as vibrations in a medium that are perceived either biochemically or electroacoustically or by a combination of the two. All vibrations can be described as a combination of three parameters—amplitude, frequency, and time (starting phase). *Amplitude* (or intensity) is the degree of displacement of the molecules in the medium; *frequency* is the rate of movement of these molecules; and *starting phase* is the point in time at which a molecule begins to vibrate (Yost & Nielsen, 1985). The force with which a piano key is struck corresponds to the amplitude or intensity of the sound, and the exact key that is hit corresponds to the frequency of the sound. Because musicians speak in terms of A, A#, B, . . . and audiologists tend to speak in terms of 440 Hz (Hertz), 466 Hz, 494 Hz, . . ., a convenient chart that provides a one-to-one translation of "letters to numbers" is useful. Figure 1–1 shows such a translation for several musical notes. The full chart is provided in Appendix I. Figure 1–1 also shows the corresponding notes on the treble cleff for that portion of the chart shown.

Near the beginning of the nineteenth century, the French mathematician Jean Baptiste Fourier (1768–1830), in analyzing heat flow, derived a series of theorems that could be applied to sound waves. Fourier's work showed that all vibrations could be represented by a series of simple vibrations (pure tones), and that one can completely characterize any sound wave by this technique if the amplitude, frequency, and starting phase are known. Indeed, if the listener is receiving the signal monaurally (through only one ear), it can be shown that only amplitude and frequency are necessary to characterize the sound. Such a technique is known as *Fourier Analysis*. However, because such a computation (based on the summing of potentially large numbers of terms in a Fourier series) can be time consuming, it was not until the development of computers that this technique became widely used. With the development of the computer, algorithms were devised which perform the tedious calculations and these have become known collectively as *Fast Fourier Transforms* (FFT).

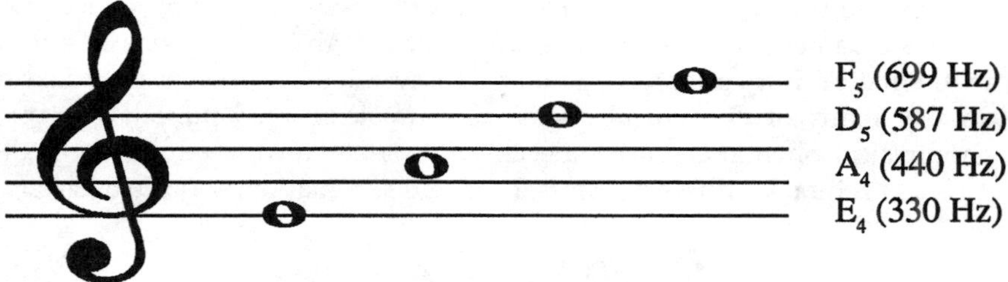

Figure 1–1. Several musical notes on the treble cleff with corresponding frequencies (in Hz). A full musical note-to-frequency chart is found in Appendix I.

Another way of looking at Fourier Analysis is that it is a technique that translates a representation of vibrations or sounds in the time domain to one in the frequency domain. Figure 1–2 shows a sound in the time domain (top) and the identical sound represented in the frequency domain. Note that the determination of frequency and amplitude becomes obvious in the frequency (spectral) domain but remains relatively obscure in the time (temporal) domain.

Fourier Analysis is certainly not the only technique that translates difficult to interpret temporal data into a spectral representation. Half a century later, the German physicist Hermann von Helmholtz (1821–1894) constructed a series of resonators which took the form of tuned brass spheres of known volumes that were coupled to short narrow tubes. Helmholtz derived a simple relationship between the volume of air in the sphere and the compliance of the air in the neck or tube of the resonator. This relationship determined the resonant or best frequency (Helmholtz resonance) of the sphere. Blowing across the top of an open pop bottle, one finds that a larger bottle will possess a lower resonant frequency than a smaller bottle. The frequency at which a given bottle resonates is its Helmholtz resonance. By holding a Helmholtz resonator up to a sound source, one can listen to the sphere and make a subjective judgment of the relative loudness at that known frequency. Performing this for a series of different sized spheres allows an individual to subjectively "draw" the spectrum of the sound.

Clearly, this partially subjective technique had limited accuracy and it was not long before the electrical analog of these spheres was employed. Using resistors and capacitors, banks of electronic filters came into popular use and indeed are still in use today, usually in a dig-

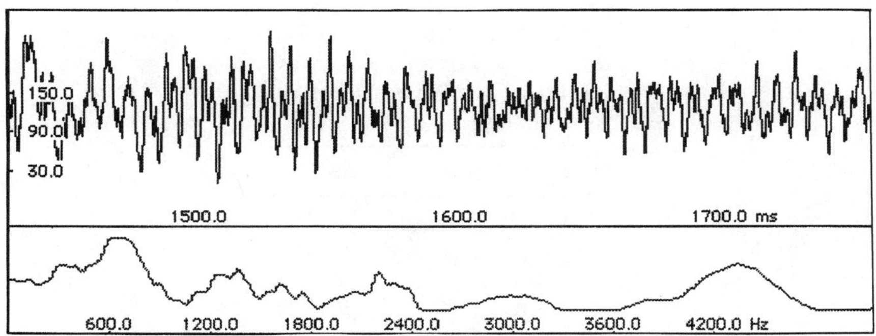

Figure 1–2. The identical sound represented in the time domain (top) and the frequency domain (bottom).

ital format. Depending on the bandwidths (range of frequencies) that characterize the filters, the type of filter, and the time constants involved, the accuracy and analysis time will vary. There are some excellent reference books on this topic and the interested reader is encouraged to pursue them. Particularly good sources are *Frequency Analysis* (Randall, 1977) and *Electroacoustics* (Hunt, 1982).

The study of how we perceive amplitude, frequency, and starting phase is called *psychophysics*. The subjective perception of amplitude or intensity is called *loudness*. There is, however, not a one-to-one correspondence between amplitude and loudness. The amplitude of a sound can increase and due to the presence of background noise, or a hearing loss, there may be no perceived loudness. However, there is never a condition, where an *increase* in one relates to a *decrease* in another. In this sense the relationship between amplitude and loudness is monotonic.

Table 1–1 shows an approximate relationship between a musical loudness judgment and physical intensity for a violinist. Note that the values have a large range, and two musicians may ascribe quite different playing intensities to a given loudness level. This can be affected by the instrument, style of music, and even musician personality.

Not all instruments have the same capability to span the range from very soft (ppp) to very loud (fff). Violins and trumpets appear to have a wide range that is relatively independent of frequency. However, the flute and French horn have a much more restricted range with a large dependence on the playing frequency. One simply cannot play a high-pitched note on the flute at a low (pp) intensity.

The subjective perception of frequency is *pitch*. Like the amplitude–loudness relationship, the frequency–pitch relationship is monotonic, but does not have a one-to-one correspondence. Unlike the

Table 1–1. Approximate Relationship Between Loudness Judgment and Physical Intensity for a Violinst

Loudness Level	dB SPL
ppp	40-50
pp	45-55
p	50-60
mf	55-70
f	70-80
ff	80-90
fff	90-110

amplitude–loudness relationship, a much smaller variance is associated with the frequency–pitch relationship. Indeed, when the frequency–pitch relationship is very well defined, we say that that individual has perfect or absolute pitch.

Because frequency is not pitch, several matching schemes have been proposed that may yield slightly different relationships. The relationship in Figure 1–1 is based on "Just Intonation," but "Equal Temperament" and "Pythagorean Tuning" relationships have been proposed which would yield slightly different conversions—usually being within 5 Hz of each other.

The primary subjective perception of starting phase is the judgment of location. This can be affected by many variables, but is only the case for binaural (two ear) hearing. It should be pointed out that the human auditory system is relatively insensitive to starting phase, and although this would make a difference in the temporal domain representation, there would be no difference in the spectral domain. Algorithms such as the FFT do indeed generate both frequency and phase spectra, but the phase spectrum can be ignored. In this condition, only amplitude and frequency are necessary to characterize the sound.

Today, both FFT and electronic filters are used in the spectral analysis of sound and vibration. For most applications these techniques work very well, and it has been the subject of much study whether the human ear functions in some way as an FFT or a filter analyzer. Many researchers have speculated on the exact nature and shape of this "internal filter." Although a study of the exact shape of this filter is beyond the scope of this book, the bandwidth characteristics (range of frequencies that can be passed by the filter) are touched upon in the loudness summation portion of this chapter.

Distortion and Harmonics

The connotation of the term *distortion* is negative and correlates with poor performance. However, depending on how it may be defined, distortion has positive attributes as well. By a very strict definition, "distortion is an undesired change in waveform" (Yost & Nielson, 1985, p. 253), but a more general and functional (albeit nonconventional) definition is the generation of energy at well-defined frequencies that were not present in the original waveform. In this sense, harmonics (and overtones) can be thought of as distortion.

Generation of energy at higher frequency multiples of a primary (an element which was present in the original signal) or a fundamental in music can be thought of as *harmonic distortion*. A system that generates distortion is called *nonlinear*. The amplitude of the harmonic distortion products defines the level of the distortion. If the amplitude is high relative to the primary or fundamental, the distortion is high. Conversely, if the amplitude is low, there is minimal distortion. However, if there is no harmonic distortion (a perfectly linear system), the fundamental note played will be a pure tone—an unpleasing beep. Figure 1–3 shows two spectra—one that has minimal harmonic distortion and one that has significant harmonic distortion (nonlinear). Both are based on the identical synthetic vowel [a] as in "father." The sound with minimal harmonic distortion is unintelligible, whereas the other is easily understood. Too high a level of distortion can be as detrimental as one that is too low.

All natural real life sound generators are nonlinear. The human voice, musical instruments, and the sounds of nature fall into this category. Harmonic distortion allows us to understand the formant or resonant structure of the human voice. Indeed, if it was not for distortion, we may never have had rock and roll.

Sam Phillips was the legendary owner of Sun Records. Like any good businessman of the day, Sam did not repair what was not absolutely mandatory. His amplifier had four vacuum tube stages and one of the tubes was broken. He simply shut down the damaged stage and turned up the gain to compensate for the remaining three stages. This set-up worked fine unless the output was high, at which time it distorted (in a well-defined manner). A recording artist named Jacky Brenston (and his Delta Cats) in 1951 recorded a song called "Rocket

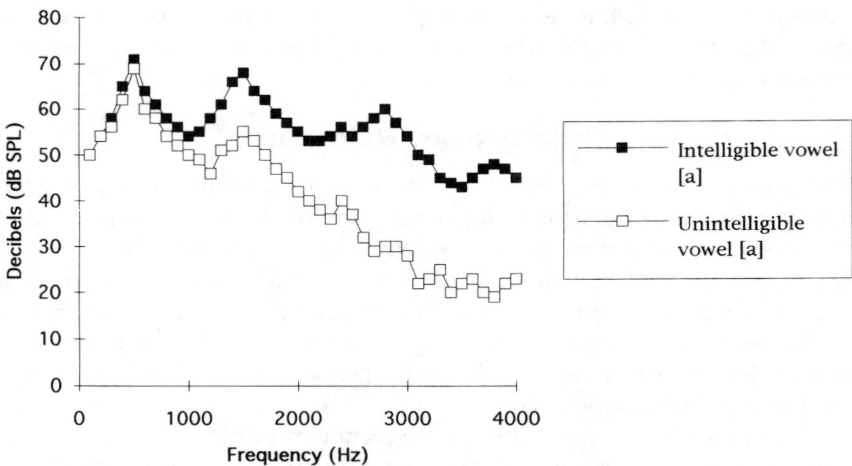

Figure 1–3. For the synthetic vowel [a] (as in "father"), the intelligibility is poorer for the one with minimal harmonic distortion (bottom). See text for explanation.

'88" at Sun Records with this amplifier set-up. The record was a commercial flop, but the "beat" on the record caused by the well-defined distortions of the malfunctioning amplifier became known as the rock and roll beat. Two years later, a young Elvis Presley re-recorded the same song.

Distortion is also something that is created by the human ear. Specifically, the inner ear creates distortion products that serve to enhance intelligibility. One of the many reasons for senior citizens having poorer speech discrimination scores relative to their pure-tone audiograms when compared with a younger population is that their cochleas are more linear (presumably caused by a stiffer basilar membrane), with a resulting loss of harmonic distortion cues.

A violinist who practices hours trying to obtain just the right tone is actually trying to alter the amplitude of the higher frequency harmonics of the fundamental note. Placing a violinist under a poorly constructed overhang in an orchestral pit will cause him or her to bow harder in order to replace some of the energy of the higher frequency harmonics absorbed by the overhang. Wrist or arm damage can occur as a direct result of the violin becoming more linear. Figure 1–4 shows the spectrum of a violin playing the identical note both under a poorly constructed overhang and with no overhang present.

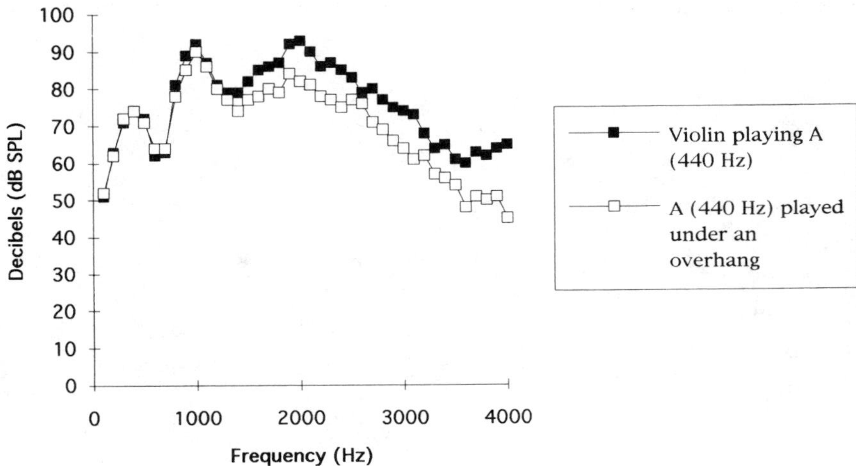

Figure 1–4. The effect on the spectrum of A_4 (440 Hz) of a poorly constructed overhang that was only 1 meter above the head of a violin player as compared with no overhang. (From "Four Environmental Techniques to Reduce the Effect of Music Exposure on Hearing," by M. Chasin & J. Chong, 1995, *Medical Problems of Performing Artists, 10,* p. 68. Copyright 1995 by Hanley & Belfus, Inc. Reprinted with permission.)

From this discussion, one can deduce that all fundamental energy of vibration has higher frequency harmonics as a result of "harmonic distortion." Indeed, perceptively, pitch is related to the difference between these harmonics and not the fundamental frequency. This phenomenon is called the *missing fundamental* or *fundamental tracking* (Roederer, 1995) and allows a listener to perceive the pitch even if the low-frequency fundamental energy is not available.

Musical instruments differ from industrial sources of vibration in one major sense: musical instruments are designed to transduce and take advantage of this high-frequency energy. A machine in a factory has most of its energy below 1000 Hz—two octaves above middle C—whereas most musical instruments have significant energy above 1000 Hz. Most industrial vibration sources have the greatest amplitude for the fundamental and successively lower amplitudes for the higher frequency harmonics. Many musical instruments have harmonics that are more intense than the fundamental. Figure 1–5 shows two spectra—a typical industrial spectrum and a spectrum of a violin playing the note A_4 (440 Hz). Note the difference in spectral shape.

The anecdote of Sam Phillips and "Rocket '88" is actually related to a different type of distortion—namely *intermodulation distortion*. Unlike harmonic distortion, which is the creation of higher-frequency energy components (usually at integer multiples of the fundamental), intermodulation distortion is the creation of lower *and* higher frequency energy

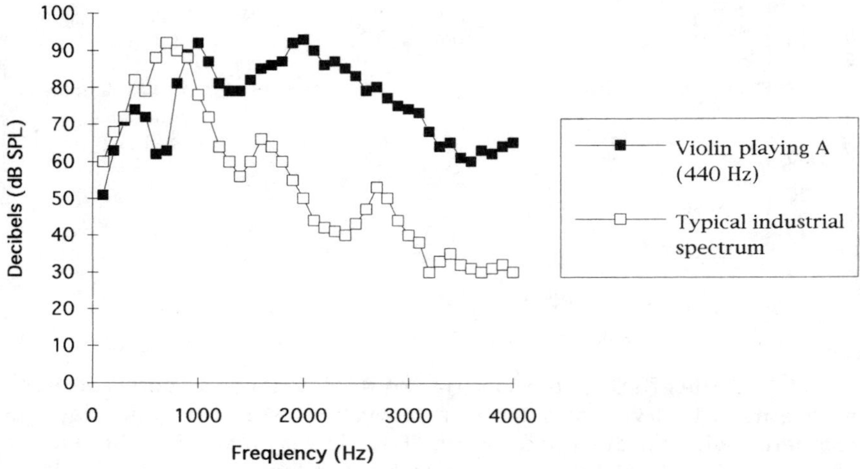

Figure1–5. The spectrum of a violin playing A_4 (440 Hz) as compared with a typical industrial noise spectrum.

components. Specifically, it is the result of a nonlinear system that yields combination tones of two or more primaries presented simultaneously. These combination tones can be related to the sum of the two primaries or, more important, to the difference between the two primaries. For example, a 700 Hz tone (f_1) and a 1000 Hz tone (f_2) may have a difference tone created at $f_2 - f_1 = 300$ Hz. This lower frequency energy at 300 Hz can be quite audible and may be viewed as either negative or positive depending on its amplitude and frequency location. Intermodulation distortion more often occurs at differences between integer multiples of the primaries. For example, if f_1 is 700 Hz and f_2 is 1000 Hz, then $2f_1 - f_2 =$ 400 Hz (or $2 \times 700 - 1000 = 400$ Hz). This third order (or cubically) distorting system is a feature of many nonlinear systems such as Sam Phillips' malfunctioning amplifier and our own auditory system.

The intermodulation distortion found in the 1951 recording of "Rocket '88" provided a beat that was to become famous. A certain level of intermodulation distortion can also be quite beneficial for understanding speech in noisy locations. Since distortion is the creation of well-defined energy components that were not present in the original waveform, these components can function as auditory cues in adverse listening situations.

Ann-Cathrine Lindblad, in studying both hard-of-hearing (1982) and normal-hearing subjects (1987) found that cubic or third-order intermodulation distortion can improve intelligibility near threshold in adverse listening situations. The basis for this finding is that there was a provision of well-defined distortion products that could be used as auditory cues in adverse listening situations.

THE HUMAN EAR

The ear is composed of several sections: the outer ear, the middle ear, and the inner ear, as well as related neurological pathways. Figure 1–6 shows the relevant anatomical features important for some of the observed characteristics of hearing. These characteristics will be discussed further.

The Outer Ear

The outer ear, the section bounded by the pinna on the lateral side and the tympanic membrane on the medial side, has two primary functions for the hearing of music. They are an amplification for higher frequency energy (the pinna effect) and the creation of a resonance in the 3000 Hz region that further amplifies higher frequency energy.

The pinna effect creates a high-frequency boost of sound energy above 2500 Hz, which gradually increases with frequency up to about 8

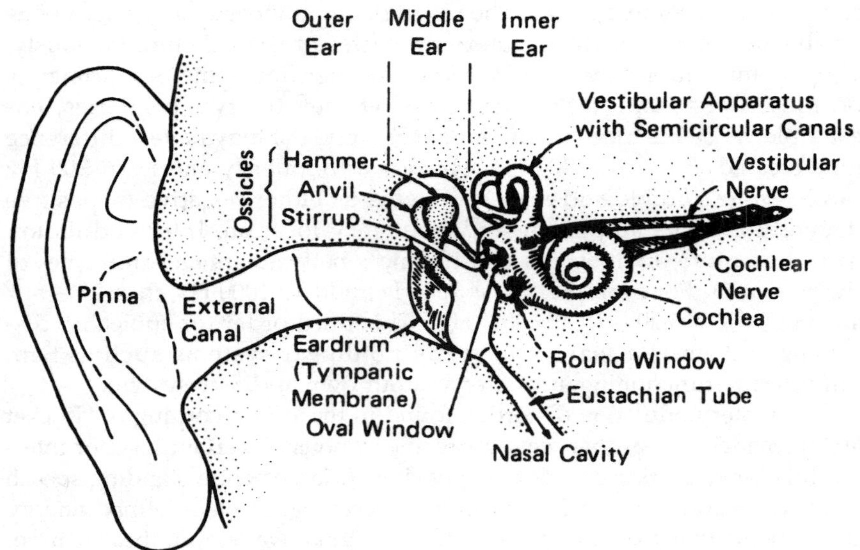

Figure 1–6. Schematic model of the ear showing some relevant anatomical features. (From *The Physics and Psychophysics of Music*, [p. 22] by J. G. Roederer, 1995, New York: Springer-Verlag. Copyright 1995 by Springer-Verlag New York, Inc. Reprinted with permission.)

to 10 decibels (dB). The physics of this effect are simple and relate to the shorter high-frequency wavelengths reflecting from the pinna back to the opening of the ear canal. In contrast, the lower frequency energy, which has longer wavelengths, are not affected by the presence of the pinna and, therefore, are not reflected back to the ear canal entrance. The "frequency–specific reflective" characteristics of sounds are described in more detail in Chapter 3.

Figure 1–7 shows this net high-frequency boost due to the presence of the pinna as well as the ear canal resonance. The total effect is also shown.

The 3000 Hz resonance (shown in Figure 1–7) is inversely related to the length of the ear canal and corresponds to a quarter-wavelength resonance. For people with very long ear canals, this resonance that is typically 15 to 20 dB tends to be at a slightly lower frequency than that of "short-eared" individuals. A wavelength resonance can be heard when blowing across the top of a length of pipe; the longer the pipe, the lower the resonant frequency.

High-frequency fundamental or harmonic energy is enhanced in intensity because of these two properties of the outer ear.

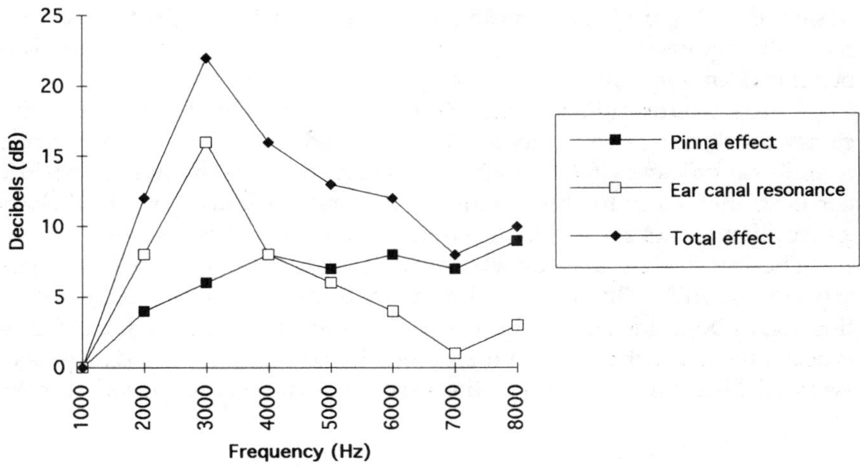

Figure 1–7. The presence of the outer ear yields a high-frequency boost. The two elements of this boost are related to the pinna effect and the ear canal resonance.

The Middle Ear

The middle ear has three major characteristics that relate to the acoustics of the sound that a person ultimately receives: impedance matching, temporary reduction of high-intensity sounds, and pressure release.

Why do we have a middle ear? The primary reason we have a middle ear is to match the characteristics of the air in the ear canal to that of the fluid in the inner ear. The middle ear can be thought of as a transformer for a train set. When we play with an electric train set we must be cautious to ensure that the 120 volts coming from the electric socket in the wall is stepped down to match the 10 to 12 volt requirements of the train set. Subsequently, all train sets come with a matching transformer (or simply a transformer) that electronically matches the wall power supply to the needs of the train set. This is known as *impedance matching*.

Similarly, the middle ear serves to match the mechanical characteristics of sound in the air to that of the fluid in the inner ear. Approximately 99% of the energy is lost when sounds go through an air–fluid barrier. This converts to 30 dB (i.e., $10 \times \log 10^{-3}$, for those who like logarithms) and can be noticed when swimming under the water while listening to someone above the surface. If there was no middle ear, our hearing sensitivity would be reduced by about 30 dB. However, as observed in Figure 1–8, the mid-frequency sensitivity is improved dramatically because of the middle ear. The effects of the middle ear are less beneficial for very low- and very high-frequency sounds.

Figure 1–9 (from Rosowski, 1991) shows a calculated middle ear efficiency for three species: human, chinchilla, and cat. Note how the human middle ear efficiency falls off above 1000 Hz. Because the human middle ear is so inefficient for high-frequency sounds, a middle ear pathology generally does not affect the high-frequency sound transmission.

The middle ear also provides for a temporary reduction of high-intensity sounds. This is related to a small muscle that is connected to the stapes bone in the middle ear, called the stapedius muscle. Such a muscle, which contracts with high-intensity sound (the stapedial reflex), serves to lessen the intensity of the person's own voice, especially for the

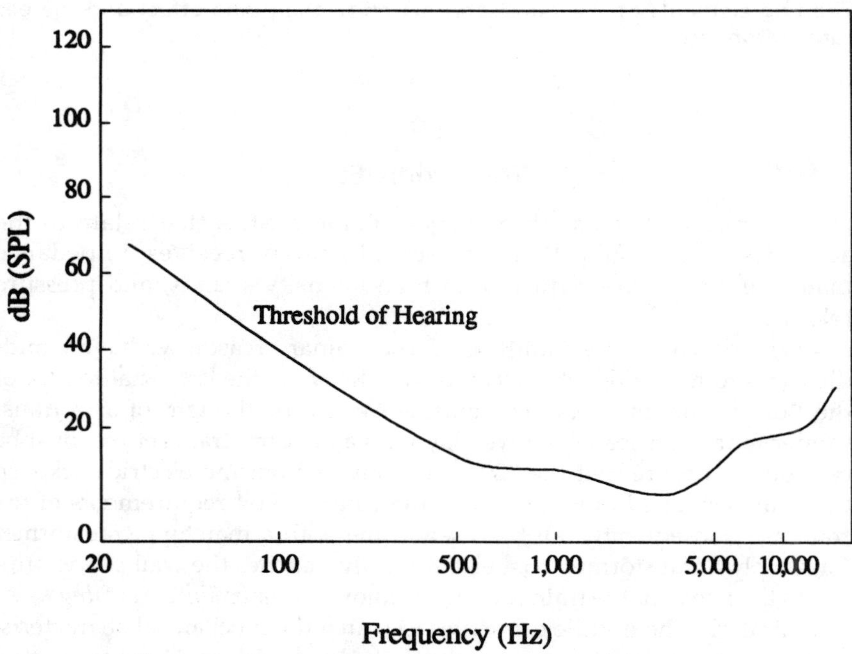

Figure 1–8. Improved mid-frequency sensitivity because of the presence of the middle-ear. (From "Loudness, its Definition, Measurement and Calculation," by H. Fletcher & W. A. Munson, 1933, *Journal of the Acoustical Society of America, 5*, p. 82. Copyright 1933 by the American Institute of Physics. Adapted with permission.)

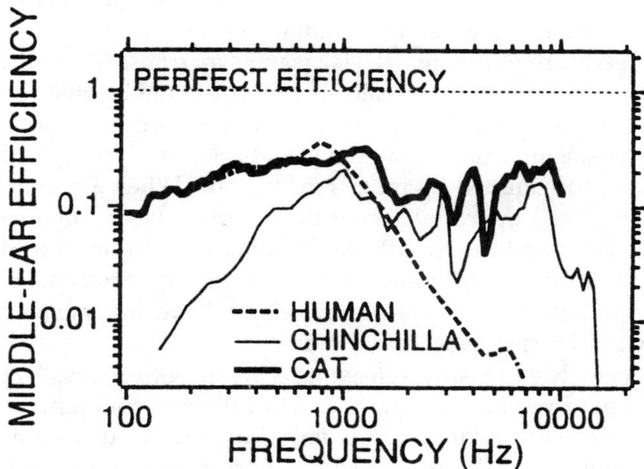

Figure 1–9. Calculated middle-ear efficiencies for three species—human, chinchilla, and the cat. (From "The Effects of External- and Middle-Ear Filtering on Auditory Threshold and Noise-Induced Hearing Loss," by J. Rosowski, 1991, *Journal of the Acoustical Society of America, 90*, p. 129. Copyright 1991 by the American Institute of Physics. Reprinted with permission.)

mid- and low-frequency sounds (Zakrisson, Borg, Liden, & Nilsson, 1980; Borg, Counter, & Rossler, 1984; Borg & Counter, 1989). However, such a neurological reflex adapts or gradually loses its function over 15 to 20 seconds. Therefore, eliciting this reflex prior to a loud sound such as a cymbal crash (by humming) may serve to lessen the damaging effects, but the duration of the effect will not be long lasting.

An upper limit for the protection from temporary threshold shift of the stapedius reflex can be greater than 20 dB in birds (Borg & Counter, 1989), and 15 dB in humans with malfunctioning stapedial reflexes due to Bell's Palsy (Zakrisson et al., 1980). Borg, Nilsson, and Counter (1983) also noted a permanent threshold shift in excess of 30 dB in rabbits with a surgically de-innervated stapedius muscle. Typical attenuations may be much less (and mostly in the lower frequencies; J. Booth, personal communication, 1995). However, even this would significantly increase the amount of time before music exposure would occur. Possibly the most important factor for why some individuals are more susceptible to hearing loss from noise or music exposure than others is because the latter have a stapedial reflex that becomes activated at a lower-intensity level, thus providing a greater amount of protection.

A third feature of the middle ear is *pressure release.* A trapped volume of air such as that found in the middle ear would not be able to respond to changes in environmental air pressure unless a "pressure valve" was utilized. The eustachian tube serves such a function. Typically, this tube is closed and is surrounded by mucus membrane. When a person yawns or swallows, the tube opens, allowing the air pressure to equalize between the environment and the middle ear. When a person has a cold, swelling occurs in the mucus membrane, thus clamping the eustachian tube shut. Pressure equalization is therefore very difficult during such a time and a temporary mild hearing loss may occur.

However, this pressure release can work both ways. Not only can the middle ear pressure be equalized with the environment, but positive middle ear pressure relative to the environment can be established with some woodwind and brass musicians. Forceful blowing against a reed or mouthpiece can cause air to be forced up through the eustachian tube into the middle ear space (Valsalva maneuver). Such a pressure differential can cause a slight temporary hearing loss that can actually benefit the musician by acting as a mild earplug (Chasin, 1989a).

Problems with the outer or middle ear (such as a cerumen or ear wax build-up, tympanic membrane perforation, middle ear infection, or a stiffening of the middle ear ossicles or bones) lead to conductive hearing losses. With a few exceptions, conductive hearing losses are medically treatable. Hearing loss related to the inner ear and associated neurological structures is referred to as a sensorineural hearing loss and, with a very few exceptions, is not medically treatable.

The Inner Ear

The inner ear (or cochlea) is a fluid-filled, snail-shaped structure about the size of the small finger nail. Running the length of the cochlea over the full two and one half spiral turns is a thin sheet called the basilar membrane. Sitting upon this membrane is the Organ of Corti which contains approximately 15,500 nerve endings or hair cells (Spoendlin, 1986). The structure of sound transduction in the cochlea is similar to that of a piano keyboard: low-frequency sounds are transduced on one end while the higher frequency sounds are transduced from the other end. Specifically, in the cochlea, high-frequency sounds are transduced by those hair cells nearer to the stapes footplate of the middle ear, while those that transduce the lower-frequency sounds are found in the innermost turns of this snail-shaped organ. There is approximately a one octave change every 1.25 mm along the basilar membrane (about 30 mm in length in adults) in the cochlea.

One quarter (about 3,500) of the nerve fibres are inner hair cells and three quarters (about 12,000) are outer hair cells (Spoendlin, 1986). Approximately 90 to 95% of inner hair cells are associated with sensory or afferent (toward the brain) neurons, whereas only 5 to 10% of the outer hair cells have afferent innervation. The outer hair cells are mostly innervated by motor or efferent (away from the brain) neurons. The cochlea presents us with a startling irregularity—the majority of the hair cells are innervated by efferent neurons and not afferent.

Until the late 1970s, the physiology of these common efferent nerve fibres was not understood, but recent research indicates that they function as a feedback loop modulating the function of the inner ear. Figure 1–10 illustrates the efferent-induced feedback change. However, others have shown that this feedback loop in the cochlea has its greatest effect for lower intensity sounds.

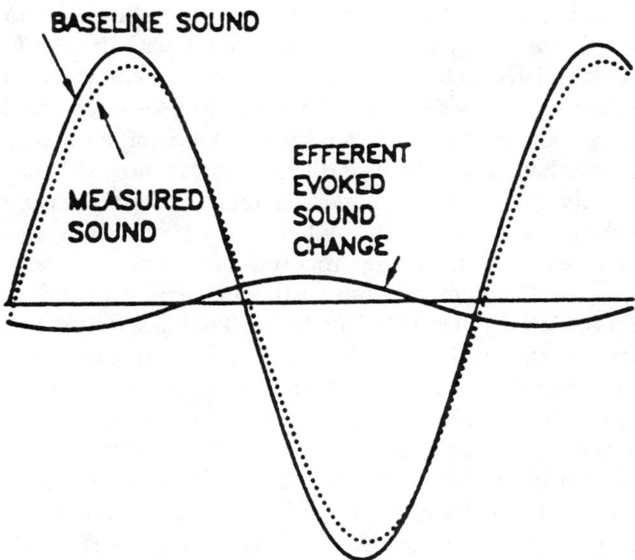

Figure 1–10. Schematic of an efferent nerve induced feedback change to the outer hair cells. (From "Effect of Efferent Neural Activity on Cochlear Mechanics," by J. J. Guinan. In *Cochlear Mechanics and Otoacoustic Emissions* [pp. 53–62], by G. Cianfrone & F. Grandori, Eds., 1986, Stockholm, Sweden: Scandinavian University Press. Copyright 1986 by Scandinavian University Press. Reprinted with permission.)

Specifically, "the outer hair cells are mostly motor rather than sensory units, amplifying the motion of faint sounds below 60 dB SPL (sound pressure level) and somehow stimulating the inner hair cells" (Berlin, 1994). These hair cells gradually lose their amplifying function for more intense sounds, with the result that while they improve the sensitivity for quiet sounds, they have no appreciable effect for more intense sounds. In this sense, outer hair cells function as a level-dependent filter.

Most people with normal hearing have emissions emanating from the outer hair cells in the inner ear. These otoacoustic emissions can be measured in the outer ear canal and have been used as indicators of hearing function (Lonsbury-Martin, Harris, Hawkins, Stagner, & Martin, 1990). Specifically, otoacoustic emissions are measurable in those individuals with normal outer and middle ears as long as there is less than about a 30 dB sensori-neural hearing loss. Although there is a large degree of variability with such measurements, recent research has indicated improved reliability utilizing otoacoustic emission delay measurements (Mahoney & Kemp, 1995).

An interesting finding is that hearing damage occurs to the outer hair cells prior to inner hair cell damage. Therefore, an abnormal otoacoustic emission test result may be observed before a measureable hearing loss is detected utilizing conventional pure-tone hearing testing. It is not clear why outer hair cells are more prone to damage than inner hair cells. One possible reason may be related to the physical location of the hair cells in the cochlea. The inner hair cells sit at the edge of a bony shelf (osseous spiral lamina) in the cochlea so they are not as affected by the motion of the basilar membrane as are the outer hair cells, which sit directly on this moving base (Lim, 1986). It is possible that this constant movement (and constant shearing by the tectorial membrane situated above the hair cells) eventually causes the outer hair cells to lose their transducing properties before the inner hair cells do.

As discussed above, the inner ear has a complicated neurological structure associated with it that includes feedback loops. In addition to this structure is the auditory cortex where much of cognition occurs. It is this central area that is related to an individual's ability to be able to attribute pitch to a sound. Approximately one person in 1,500 can perform this task with amazing accuracy (called perfect or absolute pitch) and this is thought to be related to the organization of the central structures (Bachem, 1955). People with perfect pitch generally maintain this ability despite significant cochlear damage (Langendorf, 1992).

THE SHAPE OF THINGS TO COME

Almost all professional musicians will eventually have some music-induced hearing loss. Hearing losses from noise exposure and music exposure have similar audiometric patterns. The low-frequency sensitivity is either normal or near normal, whereas sensitivity in the 3000 to 6000 Hz region is reduced. Yet, the acuity of an 8000 Hz sound is much better and like the lower frequencies can be normal or near normal. This audiometric notch, shown in Figure 1–11, is characteristic of many forms of music exposure. Yet there may be some subtle differences which will be discussed in Chapter 2.

Unlike from industrial noise exposure, a musician's hearing loss may have asymmetries where one ear is audiometrically better than the other ear. This is frequently observed in the worse left ear of the violinist or drummer, and the worse right ear of the flute player. Unlike an industrial environment, a musician's environment is rarely reverberant,

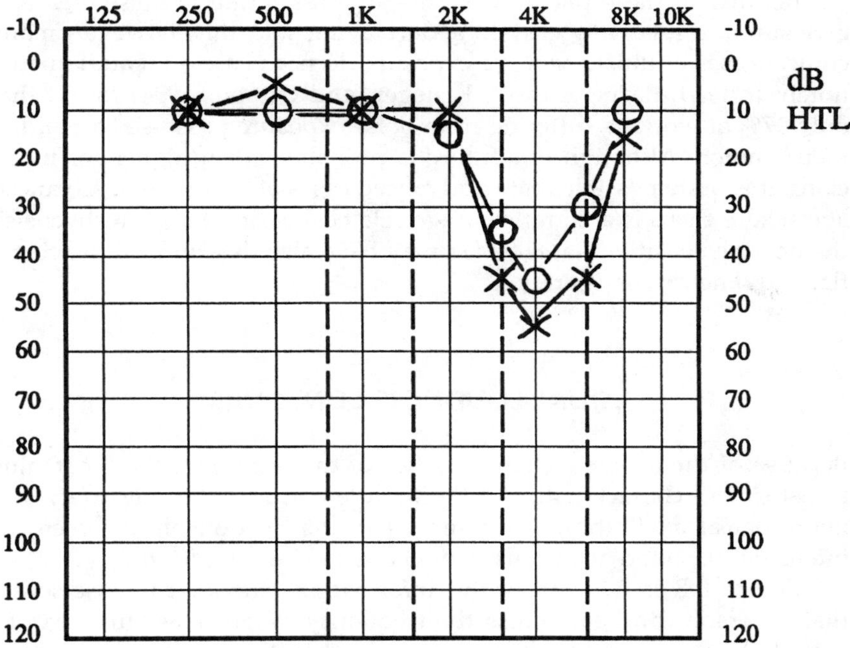

Figure 1–11. Audiogram showing a hearing loss characteristic of many forms of music exposure.

and it is this reverberation that is one of the main sources of symmetrical hearing losses among industrial workers. Another difference is that musicians who play treble instruments may have an 8000 Hz notch in their hearing that is slightly higher than the 3000 to 6000 Hz range of most industrial workers.

What are the causes of the nonmonotonic nature of music (and noise) induced hearing loss that creates an audiometric notch? Several explanations have been proposed for this notch. These include (a) a poor blood supply to the part of the cochlea that corresponds to the 3000 to 6000 Hz region (Crow, Guild, & Polvogat, 1934); (b) a greater susceptibility for damage of the supporting structures of the hair cells in this region (Bohne, 1976); (c) the orientation of the stapes footplate into the inner ear is such that its primary force vector aims toward those hair cells in this region, with the effect of eventual failure because of the constant hydromechanical action (Hilding, 1953; Schuknecht & Tonndorf, 1960); (d) permanent noise exposure has its greatest effect approximately one half octave above the peak frequency of the noise spectrum. Since all spectra are enhanced at 3000 Hz by the outer ear canal resonance, the greatest loss will be in the 4000 to 6000 Hz region (Tonndorf, 1976; Caiazzo & Tonndorf, 1977).

Because of these phenomena, hearing losses due to noise or music exposure are relatively easy to spot. Having said this, however, many clinical cases of music or noise exposure do not possess an audiometric notch. Indeed, Barrs, Althoff, Krueger, and Olsson (1994) found that only 37% of workers suffering from noise exposure possessed an audiometric notch. Although this figure is probably much higher for musicians, it is quite possible that in advanced cases of exposure or advanced age where there is a significant age-related hearing loss (presbycusis), the hearing sensitivity at 8000 Hz may have also deteriorated, leaving a flat audiometric configuration.

EQUAL LOUDNESS CONTOURS

Because of the acoustic characteristics of the outer ear, the "matching transformer" characteristics of the middle ear, and the sensitivity and neurological integration of the inner ear, the relationship between the intensities of sound at various frequencies can be complicated.

Figure 1–8 shows part of this information—the least intense sound that a person can hear across the frequency range. This curve can be thought of as an *equal loudness contour*. That is, this is a curve where all frequencies are judged to be equally loud. It typically takes an intense low-frequency sound just to be audible, and a much less intense mid-frequency sound just to be audible.

However, do all equal loudness contours have a similar bowl shape? If we were to perform an experiment where we attempted to obtain judgments on the similarities of the loudness of many tones, we would ultimately come up with a full range of contours—equally loud judgments of different frequencies. Clinically, this is not done because of time constraints, the amount of training required by the listener, and the degree of variability in the data. However, data are available from many experiments that show similar results: equal loudness contours tend to "flatten out" as the test intensity is increased.

Figure 1–12 shows this feature of flattening out. The bottom curve (threshold of normal hearing in a sound field) is very bowl shaped (identical to that found in Figure 1–8), but the bowl becomes a flattened dish at a test level of 60 dB and above. These curves have also been named after the various researchers who have studied them. The most popular alias is the Fletcher-Munson curve after Fletcher and Munson (1933), but similar data have also been obtained by Sivan and White (1933), and Stevens (1961), to name but a few. There are subtle differences and they probably relate to testing technique, equipment set-up, and subject variability. Exact values for equal loudness contours should be viewed with caution.

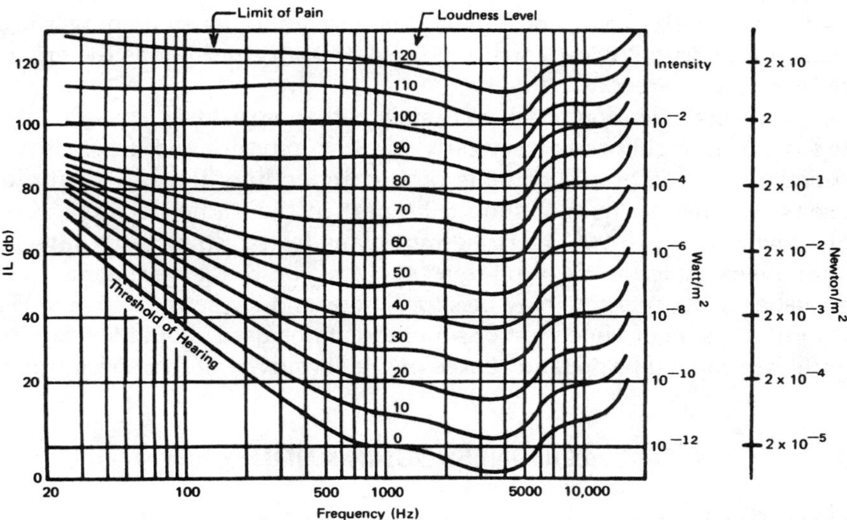

Figure 1–12. Equal loudness contours showing the flattening out feature as stimulus level is increased. (From "Loudness, its Definition, Measurement and Calculation," by H. Fletcher & W. A. Munson, 1933, *Journal of the Acoustical Society of America, 5,* p. 82. Copyright 1933 by the American Institute of Physics. Reprinted with permission.)

When hearing is tested on an audiometer, data similar to the bottom curve are used to calibrate the test machine. A reading of 0 dB on the audiometer would be a wide range of sound pressure levels depending on the test frequency. A flat "audiogram" at 0 dB, which is a graphical measure of hearing, would indicate normal hearing. A 30 dB loss in the hearing at 6000Hz (an audiometric notch), which is frequently observed in the hearing of industrial workers and musicians, implies that that individual's equal loudness contour would require a 30 dB more intense level at 6000 Hz than that of a normal hearing person. Yet if measured at a higher stimulus level, the person's equal loudness contours would tend to flatten out. This is one reason why people do not notice a mild hearing loss as long as people speak at an intense enough level.

In some sense, the typical audiogram that measures an equal loudness contour at the threshold of hearing can be thought of as an artifact. A mild loss may be viewed as completely normal if a similar equal loudness contour was instead performed at a higher level—one that would have a flattened dish shape. Only two equal loudness contours can be clinically assessed without additional training while still maintaining a high level of reliability: the minimal audibility threshold and the pain threshold. However, a person may have a very significant hearing loss and still have a normal pain threshold, so such an alternative audiogram would be rather insensitive (as well as uncomfortable). In this sense, an audiogram with a mild notch should be thought of as an early warning indicator of pathological equal loudness contours and not as the end of one's musical career.

A further extention of this reasoning is that otoacoustic emission testing can be thought of as a very early warning indicator and if our clinical function is to warn our patients of any impending damage, then otoacoustic emission testing should be part of the audiometric battery. However, as up to 90% of those musicians tested do already have an audiometric notch in the 4000 to 6000 Hz region of the audiogram, otoacoustic emission testing may be superfluous and too sensitive a test. The clinical decision of which test or set of tests to be used should be coupled with the proper interpretation based on the sensitivity of that specific test.

LOUDNESS SUMMATION

What does loudness mean to a musician and how does it change with frequency? This all relates to the bandwidth of a theoretical internal filter—a model of how the cochlea divides sound into frequency segments such as those found on the piano keyboard. Data from various aspects of auditory psychophysics indicate a specific bandwidth or range of frequencies centered around test frequencies in which responses to sound appear to be similar. Specifically, such a critical bandwidth (for loudness) is "that frequency band within which the loudness of a band . . . of sound . . . is independent of its bandwidth" (Yost & Nielsen, 1985, p. 251). That is, the loudness of a single pure tone will be judged to be equally loud as groups of two or more pure tones of similar intensity, as long as they are closely spaced. If this band of pure tones exceeds such a critical bandwidth (the bandwidth of the internal filter in the cochlea), the loudness of the sound will begin to increase. Like equal loudness contours, the critical bandwidth has been established through a series of experiments, and increases with frequency from a little over 100 Hz for the very low-frequencies to over 2000 Hz for higher frequency sounds. One critical bandwidth corresponds to a distance of approximately 0.9 mm on the basilar membrane (Moore, 1986).

All musical instruments (including the human voice) possess energy at the fundamental frequency, which is the note being played. For example, concert A has its fundamental energy at 440 Hz with no lower frequency energy. It also has harmonics at higher frequency multiples of 440 Hz such as 880 Hz and so on. The difference between these two areas of energy is 440 Hz, which is greater than the critical bandwidth for that frequency region. Even the lowest bass note will have its first harmonic at a point which exceeds the critical bandwidth in that frequency location. Thus, harmonics not only add to the richness of music but are invaluable clues to the loudness of the music.

Using the wrong ear protection can attenuate these higher frequency harmonics with not only an unfortunate loss of the beauty of music, but also of the loudness perception. Overplaying is a commonplace problem with the wrong ear protection and, as will be seen in Chapter 8, can result in wrist and arm damage.

TINNITUS

Tinnitus is defined as a perceived acoustic sensation that occurs in the absence of an external sound source. It may be classified as objective or subjective. Objective tinnitus is extremely rare and can be audible by another person in the room. This is usually related to a vascular or muscular etiology. In contrast, subjective tinnitus is heard only by the patient.

Depending on the study, up to 30% of the population may suffer from tinnitus (Coles, 1987) and 1% of patients report that it significantly interfers with daily living (Tyler, Aran, & Dauman, 1992).

Most of the research in this area pertains to developing treatment models rather than determining the etiology (Knox, 1993) and this is understandable given the wide range of possible sites of lesion covered by the one term "tinnitus." Nevetheless, there has been some progress in the development of an animal model by Pawel Jastreboff and Jonathan Hazell (Jastreboff and Hazell, 1993; Hazell, Jastreboff, Meerton, & Conway, 1993) based not only on damage to the outer and inner hair cells, but to higher neurological structures as well. Research in this area is currently concentrating on the electrical suppression of tinnitus, utilizing a well-controlled alternating current.

Other treatments of tinnitus have also appeared in the literature such as intravenous use of lidocaine (Murai, Tyler, Harker, & Stouffer, 1992), various antidepressants (Johnson, Brummet, & Schleuning, 1993), and behavior modification and psychotherapy intervention. The use of hearing aids has been shown to reduce the annoyance of tinnitus in many subjects as has the use of tinnitus maskers in a lesser number of subjects.

It should be pointed out that no single approach works well and can be considered a cure. An eclectic approach that includes elements of masking, biofeedback, psychological counseling, as well as various suppression techniques may be the most optimal clinical approach.

DIPLACUSIS

Diplacusis is a pathological matching of frequency and pitch brought about by a sensorineural hearing loss. Davis, Morgan, Hawkins, Galambos, and Smith (1950), in studying this phenomenon, noted that in a damaged region of the ear, an increase in the frequency of a sound was perceived as an increase in the loudness. The pitch remained relatively constant. Such a pitch perception problem would understandably be disasterous for a musician and can cause a note to sound flat (i.e., its pitch is perceived to be lower than it normally would be). On occasion it is this problem that causes a musician to seek professional advice and usually a significant hearing loss is apparent that may require remediation. Depending on the musical instrument, a judicious use of nonstandard ear protection may alleviate the problem to the extent that the musician can again perform.

Diplacusis can be a career–threatening problem, especially for violinists and viola players, and every effort should be made to prevent it by decreasing the potential for hearing loss.

SUMMARY

Based on a "just intonation" matching scheme, Appendix I contains a musical note-to-frequency conversion chart. This translation device allows audiologists and musicians to communicate more effectively during the assessment and the counseling phases.

Distortion, equal loudness contours, and tinnitus are common subject areas that arise. Both harmonic and intermodulation distortion products are discussed in a positive light in which their presence should be viewed as essential input to our auditory systems. Equal loudness contours, even for some with significant sensorineural hearing loss, are discussed in terms of those musicians having normal or near normal loudness perception at higher intensity levels. Therefore, musicians may not require equalization, or amplification, at higher levels.

Acoustic features of the outer, middle, and inner ears were discussed. The outer ear functions to provide high-frequency amplification. The middle ear functions to provide an impedance matching between the air in the outer ear and the fluid in the inner ear, as well as for a temporary reduction in the sound level of high intensity stimuli. The inner ear is a complex neurological system that includes a feedback path to the outer hair cells that are mostly motor, rather than sensory, units.

Tinnitus and diplacusis are two psychophysical phenomena that can be associated with sensorineural hearing loss and, depending on the severity, may pose a career-threatening injury for the musician. Prevention of hearing loss is therefore an important cornerstone to the assessment and counseling of musicians.

CHAPTER

2

Factors Affecting Hearing Loss

INTRODUCTION

Hearing losses due to noise exposure and music exposure have many similarities and in many cases cannot be distinguished. The primary method to distinguish between the two causes is the case history, which is covered in Chapter 6. Depending on the musical instrument, the environment, and those instruments in the immediate performing vicinity, one may be able to distinguish between nonmusical noise exposure and music exposure. More often than not, however, the two causes will be inseparable.

This chapter will provide an overview of those factors known to cause hearing loss, as well as those that may cause one musician to be more or less prone to hearing loss than another. Whenever appropriate, differences between the susceptibilities of musicians and nonmusicians will be discussed.

Most of the research on these factors has been performed on noise exposure rather than music exposure per se, but for all intents and purposes the results can be extrapolated to music exposure. In those few cases where this is not the case, there will be a discussion of the possible reasons.

TEMPORARY AND PERMANENT THRESHOLD SHIFTS

Most of the studies in this subject area relate to hearing loss in large-scale field studies and from experiments with animal models. The most common type of experiment is to elicit a temporary hearing loss referred to as a temporary threshold shift (TTS). As the name implies, TTS is the temporary elevation of the hearing threshold at one or more of the test frequencies and can be thought of as an early warning sign for a potentially permanent threshold shift (PTS). We all have experienced TTS after a noisy rock concert, after mowing the lawn, or even after a noisy social event. A feeling of numbness or dullness in the ears is perceived for a number of hours after the event and there may be an associated tinnitus or ringing in the ears for a period of time. If an individual's hearing was to be assessed immediately after such a noise event, a temporary sensorineural hearing loss may be found, which would typically resolve in 16–18 hours.

TTS typically occurs at approximately one half octave above the stimulus frequency and, as noted in Chapter 1, this would be in the 3000–6000 Hz region for most noise sources and for music. For very low-frequency stimuli (below 500 Hz), the region of TTS would be in the 300–750 Hz band regardless of exact stimulus frequency (Mills, Osguthorpe, Burdick, Patterson, & Mozo, 1983).

The relationship between TTS and PTS is not well defined, but it would be useful to examine some known correspondences. If a relationship was established, TTS could be used as a predictor of PTS. In 1966, the Committee on Hearing and Bioacoustics (CHABA) attempted to establish a model that would define the relationship between TTS and PTS. In the words of CHABA, "If any single band exceeds the damage-risk contours specified, the noise can be considered as potentially unsafe" (Kryter, Ward, Miller, & Eldredge, 1966).

Because of the gaps in information and lack of a firm theoretical basis, CHABA made several assumptions in order to obtain the resulting damage risk contours. One such simplifying assumption was that the recovery from TTS is related only to the magnitude of the TTS; the larger the TTS, the longer it takes to resolve. However, subsequent research demonstrated that "recovery from TTS depends on both the duration and the intensity of the noise exposure" (Melnick, 1991, p. 149).

Another implicit assumption was that intermittent noise with regular quiet periods would be less damaging than steady state noise. But how quiet do the spaces in between the noise bursts have to be for there to be a reduction in the level of damage? Ward, Cushing, & Burns (1976) developed upper limit estimates of effective quiet (a level that would produce no TTS) and these were significantly quieter than that which CHABA utilized for its damage risk contours. These are shown in Table 2–1.

Mills, Gilbert, and Adkins (1979) also calculated critical levels, which are those octave band intensities that would cause 5 dB of TTS after 16 hours. These authors summarized the results of seven earlier studies on humans of critical levels which can also be found in Table 2–1. The data from Ward, Cushing, & Burns (1976) and Mills, Gilbert, & Adkins (1979) are remarkably similar, once corrected for the difference in definition between effective quiet and critical level.

Table 2–2 shows intensity ranges (dBA) measured at the playing position of three instruments in an orchestra while these instrument sections were at rest.

Table 2–2 indicates that while the lower-frequency "quiet" levels in a typical orchestra may not be effectively quiet, sound energy above

Table 2–1. Estimates of "Effective Quiet" for Different Studies

	Ward et al. (1976)	Mills et al. (1979)	Ranges from 7 Studies (Mills et al., 1979)
250	77 dB SPL	—	—
500	76	82	75–85
1000	69	82	81–82
2000	68	78	77–78
4000	65	74	74–76
Broadband	76 dBA	78 dBA	

Table 2–2. Intensity Ranges Measured at Playing Position of Instruments in Orchestra While These Sections at Rest

	Clarinet (dBA)	Violin (dBA)	Trumpet* (dBA)
250	72–82	75–84	75–98
500	73–84	75–87	76–98
1000	69–81	71–78	70–87
2000	66–74	70–74	66–77
4000	56–62	59–65	60–67

* The wide range for the trumpet section depends on whether the French horn section was playing.

1000 Hz does achieve this criteria. Depending on the musical piece, the orchestra size, and one's exact position in the orchestra pit or stage, there may be some relief from hearing loss by the intermittent nature of music. Certainly musicians in smaller groups such as quartets would receive a greater relief from the intermittent nature of the music than would musicians in a large orchestra or rock band.

Rock bands may never achieve an effective quiet level. Even though the playing intensity is highly variable, the mean of many measurements indicates small standard deviations and thus the noise can be considered to be steady state.

Clearly, intermittence and fluctuating noise add to the difficulty in establishing damage risk criteria. The variability of the intensity of music can be thought of as "on times" and "off times," with the on times being the more intense passages and the off times being the quieter pianissimo passages. The CHABA damage risk contours (Kryter et al., 1966) utilize a relationship referred to as the "on fraction rule . . . [that] predicts that when the noise is on for half of the total period of exposure, the amount of TTS would be one-half of that which would have been produced if the noise had been continuous" (Melnick, 1991, p. 150). There have been some criticisms of this relationship but they pertain to longer on times than 2–3 minutes and for spectra with significant low-frequency energy below 1200 Hz (Selters & Ward, 1962; Melnick, 1991).

Most music sources have on time passages (mezzo forte and louder) of less than 2 minutes with most of their spectral (harmonic) energy being above 1000 Hz. As long as off times are effectively quiet, many musicians who play instruments with significant treble energy in relation to the fundamental should have less TTS according to the CHABA fraction rule. Exceptions to this are the bass and tympani players, but the relation is possibly affected by the action of the stapedius muscle, which attenuates low frequencies for these instrument group musicians.

Whether the full benefit of intermittent noise or music can be achieved by that individual or not, undoubtedly some relief is provided, but its exact magnitude cannot be precisely ascertained. "If it is possible to venture any general conclusion . . . [it is that] intermittence does reduce hazard" Ward (1991, p. 168).

The relationship between PTS and TTS is not simple. Although some individuals may appear to be prone to hearing loss from noise or music exposure as evidenced in a large PTS or long recovery time from TTS, the correlation is very low when group data are taken (Taylor, Pearson, Mair, & Burns, 1965; Henderson, Hamernik, & Sitler, 1974; Henderson, Subramaniam, & Boettcher, 1993). One can say, however, that if noise or music does not cause TTS, then it will also not cause PTS (U.S. Department of Labor, 1981; Henderson et al., 1993).

Ward (1970) suggested that an examination of recovery time from TTS may provide a better index of predicting PTS as long as the noise is high intensity and high frequency. Such a noise spectra is found commonly in the case of rock drummers and others in the immediate vicinity. A longitudinal study of these musicians may provide some reliable predictive data.

PTS and Some Models

Between 1968 and 1973 there were a number of field studies on the relationship between noise exposure and PTS (Passchier-Vermeer, 1968, 1971; Robinson, 1968, 1971; Baughn, 1973; Lempert & Henderson, 1973). Indeed, the Passchier-Vermeer, Robinson, and Baughn studies formed the basis of the 1973 U.S. Environmental Protection Agency's (EPA) Criteria Document and noted very little PTS for noise levels below 85 dBA if exposed for 8 hours per day for 40 years. It should be pointed out that this is for the average PTS measured at 500 Hz, 1000 Hz, and 2000 Hz. Although these studies had good correlation at these mid-range frequencies, the agreement was poorer for 4000 Hz, especially for the higher exposure levels.

The Lempert and Henderson (1973) study formed the basis of the National Institute for Occupational Safety and Health (NIOSH) model and is in good agreeement with the previous studies at lower exposure levels, but tended to predict a greater PTS at higher exposure levels if measured at 500 Hz, 1000 Hz, and 2000 Hz.

A more recent model is based on the International Organization for Standardization (ISO) standard R-1999 (1990) which appears to be in good agreement with the previous models. Indeed "models such as ISO R-1999 are sufficiently accurate to support the needs of most regulators, administrators, and others who need rough predictions on the effects of noise on groups of workers" (Johnson, 1991, p. 174). There are some criticisms of ISO R-1999 and these mostly revolve around the interaction between noise exposure and the effects of presbycusis (Bies & Hansen, 1990; Macrae, 1991; Bies, 1994). For younger workers (and musicians) these criticisms should not be a factor, however. At the other end of the scale, Rosenhall, Pedersen, and Svanborg (1990) showed that by age 79, there was no longer a difference between those who had been exposed to noise and those who had not. That is, eventually presbycusis becomes a much more dominant factor.

Related to the Rosenhall et al. (1990) data, an interesting feature regarding the progression of PTS over time can be seen in Figure 2–1. ISO R-1999 predicts a greater rate of increase in PTS over the first few years of noise exposure than in subsequent years. If this is indeed the case for musicians, it is imperative that there be early education regard-

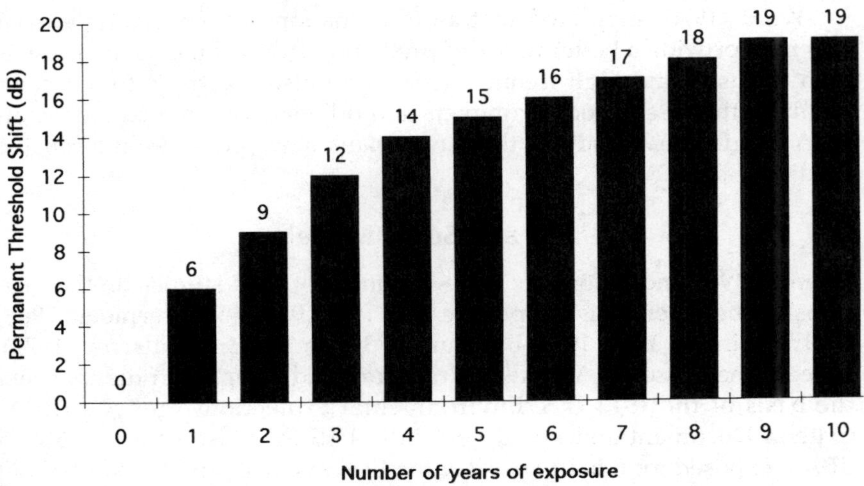

Figure 2–1. Predicted permanent hearing loss over time by the ISO R-1999 model. A greater rate of PTS is predicted over the first few years of noise exposure than in subsequent years.

ing the potential effects of music (and recreational noise). An alternative way of looking at these same data is that by the time a musician seeks audiological advice, the progression of hearing loss may have slowed and this would be useful in counseling a musician that he or she "will not go deaf."

Table 2–3 summarizes the 4000 Hz PTS of these studies at three exposure levels (85 dBA, 90 dBA, and 95 dBA).

There are no large databases for exposures levels below 85 dBA, and while some data indicate a small PTS after a number of years for exposure levels as low as 75 dBA (Robinson, 1968, 1971), and a small TTS (Mills et al., 1979), nonoccupational sources of noise and music exposure can become very significant. It would be impossible to factor these nonoccupational sources into a model with any degree of certainly or accuracy. Recreational noise is certainly one factor (Clark, 1991b; Johnson, 1991), but the long-term effects have not yet been established.

Impulse Noise and Models

Most of the models of noise-induced hearing loss are adequate for levels up to 115 dBA; however, they tend to break down for more intense impulse stimuli such as those observed with some percussion instruments. Price and Kalb (1991), and Price (1994) investigated the effects of

Table 2–3. Summary of Five Studies on Predicted PTS at 4000 Hz for Three Exposure Levels

	PASSCHIER-VERMEER	ROBINSON	BAUGHN	NIOSH	ISO R-1999
85 dBA	8	6	9	5	6
90 dBA	15	12	14	11	11
95 dBA	23	18	17	20	21

intense impulse sounds and found that the motion of the basilar membrane during the impulse sound was also important for the prediction of hearing loss (other than intensity and duration). Price (1994) notes that "at lower SPLs losses are in all likelihood largely a function of the metabolic demand on the inner ear (it gets 'tired out') and that above some spectrally dependent critical level, the loss mechanism changes to one of mechanical disruption . . . (the ear gets 'torn up')." He argues that if the basilar membrane is allowed to oscillate past the zero (atmospheric pressure) point, then more damage will be sustained by the hair cells in the Organ of Corti. If impulses possess either completely positive or completely negative pressure waves, the displacement of the middle ear ossicles cannot impart sufficient energy to create a "tearing" action to the inner ear structures.

Despite a cap pistol (at 30 cm) and two small wooden blocks (impacting at 2 cm) having almost identical peak sound pressure levels (at 150–153 dB SPL), because of the shape of the pressure wave, the small wooden blocks would cause a 25 dB permanent hearing loss but the cap pistol would only cause a 10 dB permanent hearing loss.

While there are occasional uses of cap guns and wooden blocks in popular music, we as of yet have little information on other percussive sounds that are more commonly found in music. Hitting bars or cymbals, depending on the pressure wave that is formed, as well as the peak intensity, may be more or less damaging than expected if the models presented here are used. This is an extremely important area for further research.

PTS and Exchange Rates

The damage risk contours discussed in the CHABA document refer to contours of equal risk of permanent hearing loss given a specified intensity and specified duration of exposure. That is, a relationship exists between the exposure sound level and length of exposure time.

This relationship is called the exchange rate. A 3 dB exchange rate (or 3 dB-rule) means that there is an identical risk if the sound level is increased by 3 dB, but for only half the amount of time of exposure. A 3 dB exhange rate would imply that the risk for damage doubles every 3 dB (or, equivalently, decreases by half for every decrease of 3 dB). A 5 dB exchange rate implies that risk doubles for every 5 dB increase in exposure level.

One can derive correspondences with a 3 dB exchange rate such as: the damage of a 95 dBA noise level for 8 hours is identical to the damage from 98 dBA for 4 hours, or the damage from 107 dBA for only 30 minutes. A 5 dB exchange rate would be more conservative: 95 dBA for 8 hours is an equivalent risk as 100 dBA for 4 hours, or 115 dBA for only 30 minutes. Thus, a 5 dB exchange rate would predict a lower risk than a 3 dB exchange rate.

The relationship of the PTS due to steady state noise with that of fluctuating noise is complicated, but some researchers (Martin, 1976; Robinson, 1976) have argued that fluctuating noise (such as that found in many types of music) can be equally hazardous as a steady state noise of "equal energy." Proponents of the equal energy hypothesis would advocate a 3 dB exchange rate.

However, many TTS experiments and researchers, such as Ward (1976), have argued that noises that produce equal amounts of TTS are equally damaging. Proponents of this point of view would advocate a 5 dB exchange rate.

Embleton (1995), in reporting on the results of an International Institute of Noise Control Engineering Working Party paper, concluded that "the scientific evidence is that 3 dB is probably the most reasonable exchange rate for daily noise exposure. Statistically it is also a good approximation for the results of many epidemological studies relating to intermittent exposures, even though these show considerable spread about any mean curve" (p. 18).

It should be emphasized that these exchange rates are meant only to summarize data and they can be an oversimplificaton (Ward, 1976). Indeed, Johnson (1973) noted that as a convenient data summarizing tool, the 5 dB exchange rate seems to be appropriate for hearing losses in the mid frequencies (500 Hz to 2000 Hz) and the 3 dB exchange rate is more appropriate for 4000 Hz. Finally, Ward (1974, 1982) points out correctly that the effects of noise exposure are caused by dosage and not merely by sound level.

MODELS AND MUSICIANS

While these models are not intended for use with individuals, general predictions can be made for groups of workers, assuming well-defined criteria such as years of exposure and intensity level. How then do these models relate to musicians? A related question concerns the sound levels that musicians are exposed to.

Spectral Shape

Lebo, Oliphant, and Garrett (1967) found that the spectral shape of symphony orchestras was fairly flat from 500 Hz up to 4000 Hz, but that rock and roll music had most of its energy between 250 Hz and 500 Hz. However, these measurements were made at the back of an auditorium. Rintelmann & Borus (1968) noted that the rock and roll spectrum, if measured at a distance of 5 feet, was flat up to 2000 Hz with a rolloff above that. More recently, Hétu & Fortin (1995) found peak levels in discoteques were in the 63 Hz region. Flottorp (1973) noted that the spectra from different orchestras were "remarkably equal" and were in good agreement with previous studies. He did find more high-frequency energy than previous studies for his pop music measurements. Flottorp noted that "the sound pressure level in octaves above 4000 Hz depend very much upon the distance from the loudspeakers, because the crowd of young people absorbs much of the energy in the highest frequency range" (p. 346). At the rear of a dance floor, the sound levels can be from 5 dB (for the low-frequency sounds) to 14 dB (for the high-frequency sounds) less intense than at the position of the performer. This, of course, depends also on the reverberation characteristics of the room. This phenomenon is discussed in more detail in Chapters 3 and 7.

Figure 2–2 shows average spectra from 10 rock and roll bands, as well as data from Lebo et al. (1967), Rintelman and Borus (1968), and damage risk contours from CHABA for continuous noise and for noise with an "on fraction" of 0.65 (the music is on for 65% of the time and there is effective quiet for 35% of the time).

Spectral Intensity

The intensity range of orchestras varies depending on the piece of music being played, the performance hall and its acoustical condition, the preferences of the conductor, and the techniques of the individual musicians. Perhaps the most intense piece of classical music is Wagner's Ring Cycle. Camp and Horstman (1992) found prolonged levels in excess of 110 dBA in some parts of the orchestra during the more intense movements of this piece (specifically the Götterdämmerung movement). In addition, they found that some musicians were receiving in excess of 187% of their daily noise dose (based on an 8-hour day and 90 dBA fence). Jansson and Karlsson (1983) found that depending on the seating position within the orchestra, musicians achieved their maximum safe

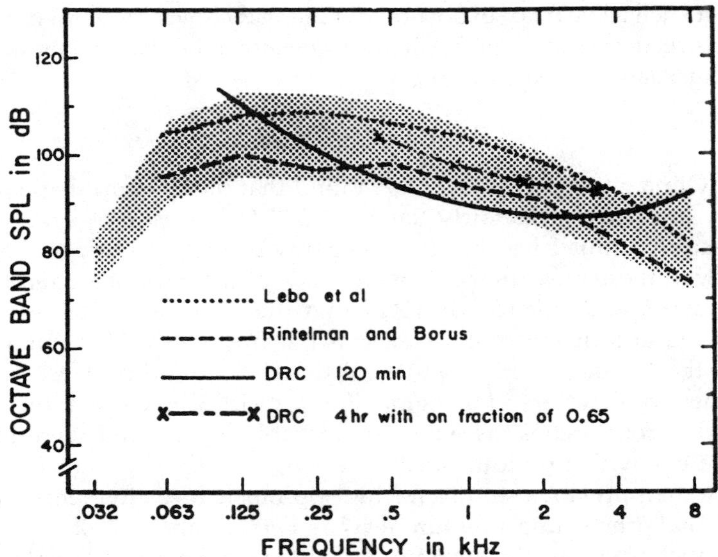

Figure 2–2. Average spectra for ten rock-and-roll bands as well as data from Lebo et al. (1967), Rintelman & Borus (1968), and damage risk contours from CHABA. (From "Hearing Loss in Rock-and-Roll Musicians," by C. Speaks, D. Nelson, & W. D. Ward, 1970, *Journal of Occupational and Environmental Medicine, 12*, p. 217. Copyright 1970, by American College of Occupational and Environmental Medicine. Reprinted with permission.)

weekly dose of exposure after only 10–25 hours of playing. McBride et al. (1992) found other excessive results for trumpet players performing Mahler's Ninth Symphony (112 dBA and 160% of their daily dose). Chasin and Chong (1991) found levels of 126 dBA, measured at the right shoulder of a piccolo player at Canada's National Ballet during a relatively quiet etude.

The intensity ranges in pop and in rock-and-roll bands tend to be rather uniform since the output is usually controlled by the sound engineer, but sound levels in excess of 120 dBA routinely have been measured (Hétu & Fortin, 1995). With the advent of lower distortion amplifiers, sound engineers are able to increase the volume further without the previous concerns of audible distortion.

Other types of popular music tend to be less intense, such as jazz, blues, and country and western. Typical intensity measurements of these performances have been measured at 80–101 dBA on stage. Cultural music, such as Japanese drum bands, has been measured at 125 dBA (Chasin, 1995a).

Axelsson and Lindgren (1978a, 1981), Westmore and Eversden (1981), Karlsson, Lundquist, and Olaussen (1983), Johnson (1985), and Royster-Doswell, Royster, and Killion (1991) found PTS in musicians; incidence in classical musicians has been shown to be up to 52% and that of rock/pop musicians, up to 30% (Hart, Geltman, Schupbach, & Santucci, 1987).

MUSICIANS AND TTS

Jerger & Jerger (1970) found that eight of ten rock musicians who had their hearing measured prior to and one hour after a performance had TTS. Speaks, Nelson, and Ward (1970) measured the hearing of 25 rock musicians prior to, at 20 minutes, and again at 40 minutes after a performance and found only 7–8 dB of TTS in the higher frequencies. However, they point out that "shifts greater than 7 to 8 dB could have occurred and then recovered to this low level during the 20 to 40 minute period before post exposure audiograms were obtained" (p. 217). Dey (1970) exposed listeners to disco music at sound levels of 100 and 110 dB SPL from 5 to 120 minutes. The measured TTS after two minutes post exposure (TTS_2) was up to 40 dB. He noted that based on the damage risk criterion, "the data indicate that, after listening for 2 hours to such music at 100 dB, two persons in 100 would recover far too slowly, whereas at 110 dB, 16 per cent would be adversely and probably permanently affected" (p. 469). More recently, Yassi, Pollock, Tran, and Cheang (1993) found that 81% of their subjects had TTS up to one half hour after the rock concert, and 76% showed continued TTS even after one hour.

In many of these studies, the amount of measured TTS was small and one would tend to be conservative of one's concerns for future PTS (see, for example, Hétu & Fortin, 1995); however, it should be pointed out (as discussed in Chapter 1) that a conventional pure-tone audiogram is limited in its scope. Otoacoustic emission testing is one alternative assessment procedure that may indicate pathology before it is observed in a conventional pure-tone audiogram (Attias et al., 1995). High resolution Békésy audiometry is another. West and Evans (1990) discussed this test, which indicates that post exposure frequency resolution can be degraded by up to 15% despite observing no measureable TTS. Pang-Ching (1982), in assessing school band directors, noted no measureable TTS and sound levels were below those necessary for initiating a hearing conservation program. However, after years of teaching, the music directors had hearing sensitivities that were 15 dB worse than those who were not subject to noise/music exposure.

TTS and Subjective Factors

A major difference between noise and music exposure is that music is presumably enjoyable. This preference for music is the source of some interesting findings with respect to TTS.

Hörmann et al. (1970, cited in Lindgren & Axelsson, 1983) studied the emotional effects on TTS at 4000 Hz. One group of subjects was given a 95 dBA noise for 30 minutes as a "reward" for performing a task and another group was given the same noise as a "punishment." The TTS for the punishment group was 18.1 dB but that for the reward group was only 12.8 dB.

Axelsson and Lindgren (1978a) found that TTS was less among rock musicians than in researchers in the audience who were performing dosimetry. Some of those performing the research found the music to be above their tolerance level and distasteful. They also found that whereas 43% of classical musicians seemed to have PTS, only 13% of pop musicians had a hearing loss. They attributed this to the finding that pop musicians were happier with their music than classical musicians who were compelled to play music they did not like.

Schönfeld (1979, cited in Lindgren & Axelsson, 1983) found that both TTS and time of recovery from TTS were greater in those who found an intense test noise unpleasant as opposed to those who were accustomed to it.

Lindgren and Axelsson (1983) studied 10 subjects exposed to noise and music of equal intensity, frequency, and time distribution characteristics. Although 4 out of the 10 subjects showed identical TTSs, the other 6 subjects showed less TTS to the music than to the noise. However, those subjects who had less TTS from music became more susceptible to TTS from music in subsequent test sessions. The authors attributed this to increasing boredom with the same test stimulus.

Swanson, Dengerink, Kondrick, and Miller (1987) found additional supportive evidence. They compared two groups of subjects: those who liked pop/rock music and those who did not. The group who liked the music had less TTS than those who disliked it. In addition, the group who liked music had less TTS from the music as compared to that from an equivalent noise spectrum. Finally, for the group who disliked the music, there was more TTS from the music than from the noise.

Axelsson, Eliasson, and Israelsson (1995), in performing a follow-up for a longitudinal study of pop/rock musicians, found that despite an average playing time of 26 years, 63% still had normal hearing and another 15% had only a very mild (less than 25 dB HL) hearing loss in the higher frequencies. They suggested that this lack of susceptibility to music energy that would cause PTS among industrial workers (according to models such as ISO R-1999) may be related to muscle proteins in the outer hair cells. These proteins have been suggested as an explanation for auditory toughening. This phenomenon (also referred to as the *training effect*) will be discussed later in this chapter.

There seem to be an ever increasing number of Broadway-like shows that run for a number of years where musicians are required to play the same songs eight times a week for years. Chasin (1995b) measured the TTS of three musicians after an initial performance and again after the 300th performance of the very same set of musical pieces. TTS increased by 6 dB to 8 dB after the 300th performance and this was statistically significant ($p < .01$). Boredom does result and, as suggested by Lindgren & Axelsson (1983), may increase performers' propensity for TTS.

Although we have little physiological evidence to explain these findings, the answer may be related to the efferent neurological pathways and the physiology of the outer hair cells in the cochlea (Axelsson et al., 1995). In addition, Axelsson and Lindgren (1978b) felt that there may be a change in the circulation in the inner ear on a hormonal basis if music was felt to be beautiful versus terrible. Muchnick, Hildesheimer, & Rubinstein (1980) found that emotional stress in guinea pigs created increased levels of catecholamines that may reduce the level of available oxygen in the cochlea. Reduced oxygen levels (anoxia) in the cochlea has been suggested as a mechanism for TTS (Lawrence, Gonzales, & Hawkins, 1967; Hawkins, 1971).

AUDITORY TOUGHENING OR THE TRAINING EFFECT

First noted by Miller, Watson, and Covell (1963), *auditory toughening* or the *training effect* is the auditory system's ability to modify its susceptibility to damage from noise, depending on previous exposures. Specifically, when the auditory system is "toughened" by nondamaging exposure to noise for a number of days, ensuing hearing loss as a result of a damaging level of spectrally similar noise is *less* than that which would occur if there was no previous toughening.

This phenomenon has been observed for PTS in a wide range of mammals as well as for TTS among teenagers (Miyakita, Hellstrom, Frimansson, & Axelsson, 1992). Figure 2–3 indicates that, after a toughening or training of the ear for 10 days to a 500 Hz band of noise, (even after a 5-day period of recovery), a smaller PTS was found than in chinchillas that were not toughened.

However, this experiment was for chinchillas that were toughened and later exposed to high levels of the same noise (e.g., 500 Hz). Subramaniam, Henderson, & Spongr (1991) examined the effects on a low-frequency toughening (500 Hz) but a high-frequency exposure (4000 Hz). In this case, the reverse result was obtained—the toughening actually *increased* the PTS over that of the nontoughened or control group.

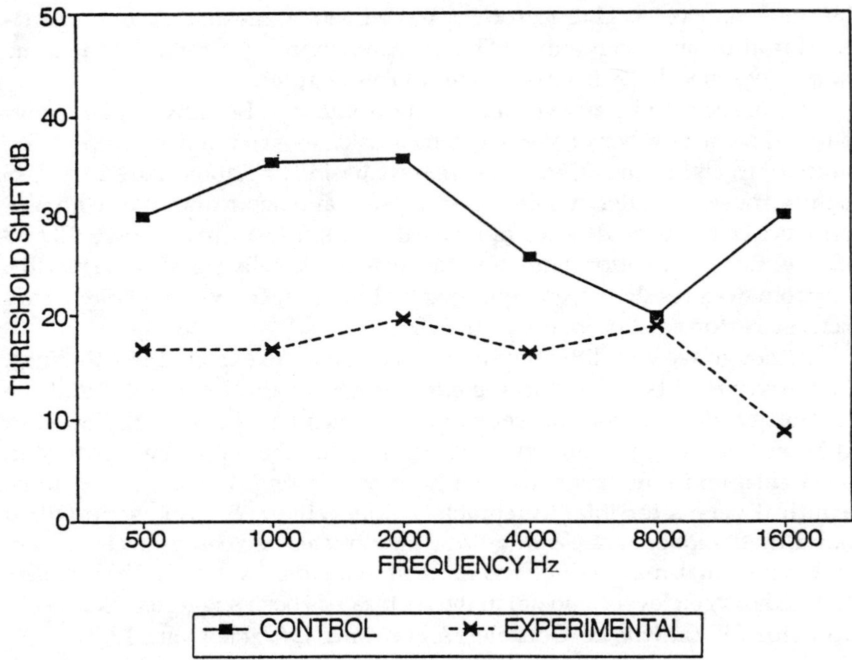

Figure 2–3. The difference in PTS between the experimental group that received 10 days of "conditioning" exposures, and a control group after a 48 hour exposure to 500 Hz at 106 dB SPL. (From "Effect of 'Conditioning' Exposures on Hearing Loss From Traumatic Exposure," by P. Campo, M. Subramaniam, & D. Henderson, 1991, *Hearing Research*, *55*, p. 197. Copyright 1991 by Elsevier Science, Inc. Reprinted with permission.)

In summary, it seems that if the nondamaging toughening stimulus is the same as the more traumatic one presented later, then there will be some protection from this effect. However, if the toughening stimulus is low frequency and the tramatic one is high frequency, then the high frequency effect may exacerbate the hearing loss.

The physiology of auditory toughening or the training effect is not well understood. Possible explanations may be related to the effects of the efferent neurological pathways and the effects of the presence of proteins in the outer hair cells. More research on this topic is required.

Musicians frequently ask the question: "Should I wear ear protection when I practice as well as when I perform?" The answer is certainly not clear, but as a general rule the answer is yes. If wearing ear protection during a solo practice session decreases the auditory system's ability to be toughened, however, then such advice may be not be completely correct. These musicians should be counseled regarding the auditory toughening data in the literature.

If a musician is exposed in an orchestra to the identical set of spectra that he or she practices at home at a less intense level, then practicing without ear protection (and performing with ear protection) may be advisable. This may be the case with a violin player who is surrounded by other violinists in a large string section. However, if this same violinist sits in front of the tympani or cymbal during performances, then ear protection is recommended for both practice sessions and performances.

Again, the appropriate clinical approach when only part of the information is known is to educate the musician conveying as much of the technical data as possible, and creating an educated consumer.

HEARING LOSS AND GENETIC FACTORS

Some studies in the research literature find evidence for an increased probability of hearing loss based on genetic factors related to eye color and sex.

Robinson (1988) found weak statistical evidence that eye color is related to hearing loss, but this is only for certain frequencies and the available sample sizes are small. Similar results previously had been found by Carter (1980), and by Carlin and McCrosky (1980). Generally, blue-eyed people were found to be more susceptible to hearing loss including from noise exposure than those with more melanin content in their eyes. Cooper (1994), in commenting on Robinson's work, found that most of Robinson's groups had statistical sampling problems that limit the validity of the conclusions. Nevertheless, Henselman et al. (1995), in studying U.S. Army soldiers, found that a significant difference in hearing levels "among the race groups with black soldiers having the most sensitive hearing and white soldiers having the poorest" (p. 382).

Cooper (1994) did, however, find that older women generally have poorer low-frequency hearing sensitivity and this may be related to estrogen and its relationship to metabolic presbycusis. At higher frequencies, Cooper noted that men had worse hearing thresholds than women, when matched for age. Berger, Royster, and Thomas (1978) also found that men had worse hearing thresholds than age-matched women when exposed to equivalent levels of noise over a number of years. Johnson (1991) attributed much of this difference to the level of nonoccupational noise exposure that men are subject to relative to that of women.

Henderson et al. (1993) noted that although genetic factors such as eye color and sex are significant in well-controlled studies, they account for only a small fraction of the variability in studies on hearing loss.

SMOKING AND HEARING LOSS

A small, but growing body of research is attempting to answer the exact nature of the interaction between hearing loss and an increased carbon monoxide level such as that found with smoking (see, for example, Chung, Wilson, Gannon, & Mason, 1982; Prince & Matonoski, 1991; and Barone, Peters, Garabrant, Bernstein, & Krebsbach, 1987). However, no definitive study provides conclusive evidence. This is probably related to the fact that those who smoke also have other physiological problems that may alter their susceptibility to hearing loss from noise exposure. Further, interactions exist that (depending on the factors and their levels) may increase or decrease one's propensity for hearing loss.

There is evidence that cardiovascular function (Sanden & Axelsson, 1981) and overall physical fitness (Ismail et al., 1973) can affect the propensity for hearing loss. Sanden and Axelsson found shipyard workers with greater increases in heart rate and blood pressure when working hard had the greatest hearing losses. Ismail et al. studied the degree of TTS initially and after these same subjects completed an eight-month physical training program and found that after the training program there was significantly less TTS.

Vittitow, Windmill, Yates, and Cunningham (1994) discussed two physiological processes in order to explain the interaction between noise exposure and poor oxygen supply to the cochlea such as that observed in some studies with smokers. The first is metabolic exhaustion and this "occurs when a hair cell [in the cochlea] fails to convert nutrients and expel waste in accordance with the stress demands placed upon it" (p. 347). When nutrients such as oxygen are not adequately supplied, hair cell damage occurs. The other process is vascular (Lawrence et al., 1967; Hawkins, 1971); noise may damage the vascular structures of the cochlea, thereby cutting off the oxygen supply route to the hair cells.

Hétu, Phaneuf, and Marien (1987), in reviewing some studies on the acute and chronic effects of carbon monoxide, found reduced performance on auditory perception tasks and concluded that the major site of lesion was the auditory cortex. Patchett (1992) found that inhalation of oxygen during noise exposure reduces TTS.

Hearing loss from noise exposure is undoubtedly related to a combination of the these processes (and sites of lesion) and indicates that excessive levels of carbon monoxide and/or lower levels of oxygen in the bloodstream would increase one's susceptibility to noise exposure. However, Dengerink, Trueblood, and Dengerink (1984) found that the effects of smoking and cold temperatures *decreased* one's susceptibility to hearing loss. They argued that both of these factors cause a *peripheral* vasoconstriction, thereby increasing the blood flow to more central locations such as the cochlea. Dengerink, Lindgren, Axelsson, and Dengerink

(1987) also found that exercise *and* smoking in noise decreased one's susceptibility to hearing loss as compared with a nonsmoking, nonexercising group. It was argued that more blood supply was available to the central locations such as the cochlea of the smokers because of the peripheral vasoconstriction of this group. In this same vein, they also found that lower body temperature decreased one's susceptibility to noise exposure.

These findings are not necessarily contradictory. Simply stated, if there is less oxygen and/or more carbon monoxide (from smoking) available to the cochlea, there will be an increased susceptibility to noise exposure. The above studies support the contention that factors affecting the cardiovascular system may have a major effect on the auditory system. In summary, to reduce the propensity for noise exposure, if people smoke, then they should make sure their cardiovascular system is healthy.

Because many smokers do have associated cardiovascular problems and tend to have more overall health problems, they should be counseled to stay away from damaging noise and music, or at least to take extra precautions to reduce the exposure.

The proper question should be: "Are people who smoke more prone to hearing loss?" and not "Does smoking contribute to hearing loss?" The answer to the first question is probably in general yes, but we don't have enough evidence yet to answer the second question.

SUMMARY

Most studies on the characteristics of hearing loss from noise or music exposure come either from large-scale field studies or from animal models. Efforts to relate TTS to PTS have met with limited success because of gaps in our knowledge as well as not having a firm theoretical base. Assumptions have therefore been made to bridge this gap. One assumption is that intermittent noise exposure with quiet periods are less damaging than constant steady state noise. Data based on the spectral characteristics of various sources of music indicate that indeed many forms of music exposure have periods that are sufficiently quiet to provide some relief to the music. The only exception may be amplified rock music.

Several models of PTS were compared. The ISO R-1999 model is considered to be accurate enough for industrial noise exposure for the requirements of most regulators. However, because of the effect of subjective factors, spectral intermittency, and the potential effects of auditory toughening, it is currently difficult to establish equivalent models for music exposure.

Genetic factors, such as eye color, and sex, are known to alter one's susceptibility to hearing loss as are factors relating to general health and smoking.

CHAPTER 3

Development of Acoustic Principles

INTRODUCTION

This chapter will provide a technical basis for the understanding of subsequent chapters of this book. Specifically, the chapters on the acoustics of musical instruments (Chapter 4), ear protection (Chapter 5), room acoustics (Chapter 7), and environmental modifications (Chapter 8) will utilize many of the principles and approaches developed here.

No previous technical knowledge of acoustics is necessary, but many similarities will be found here with hearing aid acoustics as well as the study of speech production. This chapter will introduce two equations (Figures 3–4 and 3–8). These equations are merely convenient tools with which to summarize those factors that affect the resonant frequency and they should be viewed as such.

The following six acoustic phenomena are not mutually exclusive, and the description for the behavior of one may relate to that of another. The chapter outline, based on these six phenomena, is as follows:

1. resonance
    - quarter wavelength resonators
    - half wavelength resonators
    - mechanical and Helmholtz resonators
2. damping

3. standing waves and vibrato
4. acoustic transformer effect
5. high-frequency reflectivity and impedance
6. sound directivity.

RESONANCE

All tubes, chambers, and cavities possess best frequencies, which are amplified by an enclosed space or structure. Examples of resonance can be found in human speech, every musical instrument, many hearing protectors, and even a vibrating sensation in one's automobile. *Resonance* is defined as the oscillation of an electrical, mechanical, or acoustic system at a certain frequency that requires relatively little energy. Figure 3–1 shows a set of resonances for a typical behind-the-ear hearing aid.

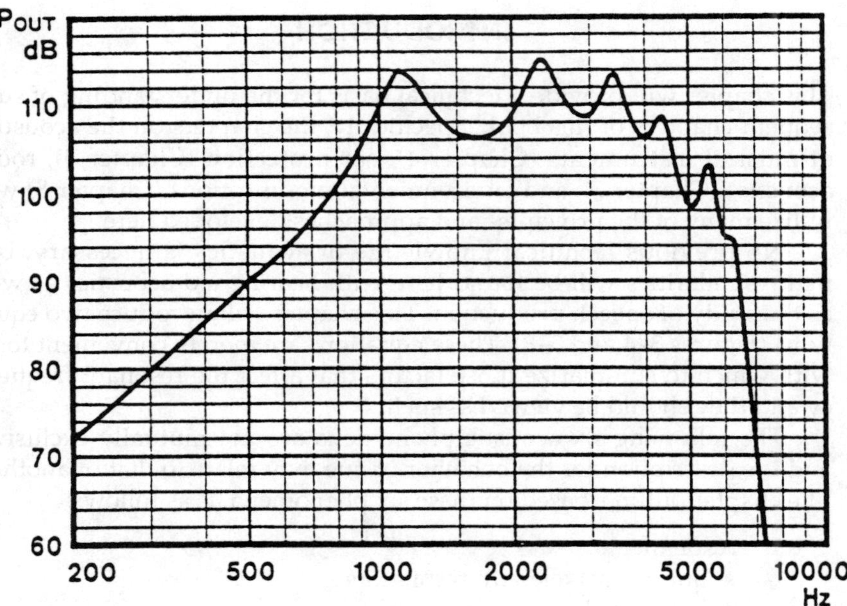

Figure 3–1. Resonances for a typical behind-the-ear hearing aid. (Courtesy of Unitron Industries Ltd.)

The resonant peak near 1000 Hz is the result of a minimum amount of blockage of the sound energy by the charcteristics of the hearing aid. In contrast, sound energy at 1500 Hz (being "off resonance") is not transduced through the system well and would subsequently not be as intense as the 1000 Hz sound energy.

This example emulates two different types of resonances—wavelength resonances and mechanical resonances. The first, third, and fifth resonant peaks are related to the hearing aid/ear mold tubing that couples the hearing aid to the hearing aid user's ear. These are *wavelength resonances.* The second and fourth resonant peaks are mechanical and electrical in nature and correspond to the charcteristics of the hearing aid receiver (loudspeaker).

Wavelength resonances, as the name implies, are created by interference patterns caused by sound waves inside the tube or "waveguide." Figure 3–2 shows such an interference pattern (of displacement amplitudes) caused by wave compressions and rarefactions travelling from one end of the tube to the other, interacting with the reflected waves travelling in the other direction. Such an interference pattern is called a standing wave, because it appears to be stationary in space. In actuality, there is significant movement, and each tube has characteristics that define where the nodes and antinodes of the standing wave are.

Nodes are physical locations in a tube where there is virtually no air particle movement. In a vibrating string, nodes are those locations that have no vibration. Placing a finger at a node on a violin string, for example, will have minimal effect. In contrast, antinodes (or loops), as the name implies, are locations with a maximum amount of air particle (or string) movement. Placing a finger at an antinode position on a violin string will significantly attenuate the sound.

Do all tubes behave identically with the same set of nodes and antinodes in their standing wave pattern? The two factors that determine

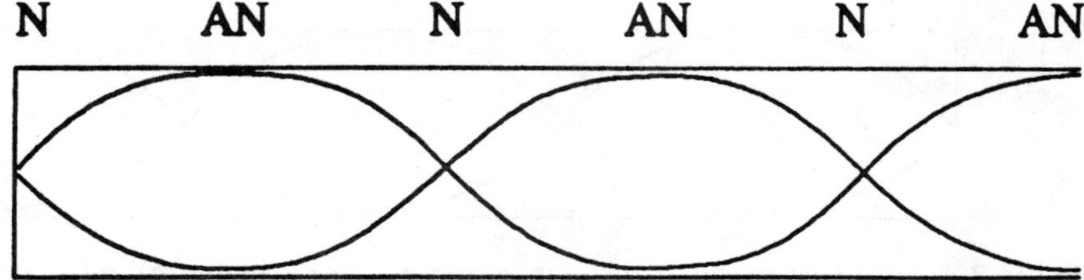

Figure 3–2. Interference pattern (standing waves) of a quarter wavelength resonator. N = node; AN = antinode.

the pattern are the effective length of the tube or string and the boundary conditions of the tube or string. *Boundary conditions* pertain to the nature of the end points. The tube shown in Figure 3–2 is "closed" at one end and "open" at the other. This tube is actually a schematic drawing of a typical behind-the-ear hearing aid whose resonant pattern is shown in Figure 3–1. It can also represent the resonant pattern of many musical instruments.

The longest wavelength (i.e., lowest frequency) that can exist in such a tube is shown in Figure 3–3a. As can be observed, this pattern corresponds to exactly one quarter of the full wavelength. The boundary condition for tubes that are closed at one end and open at the other end defines a *quarter wavelength resonator*. Figures 3–3b and 3–3c show the second and third modes of resonance of such a tube. In all cases, there must be a node (N) at the closed end and an antinode (AN) at the open end.

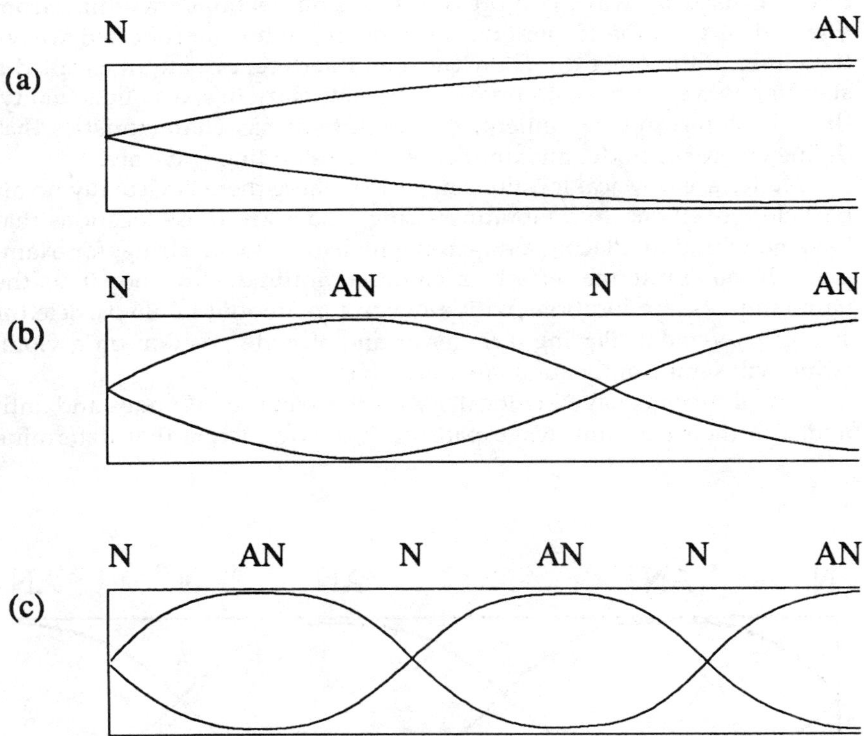

Figure 3–3. (a) First mode of resonance of a quarter wavelength resonator (i.e., the lowest frequency resonance); (b) second mode of resonance of a quarter wavelength resonator; (c) third mode of resonance of a quarter-wavelength resonator. N = node; AN = antinode.

Examining Figures 3–3a, 3–3b, and 3–3c, it is noted that while Figure 3–3a corresponds to ¼ of a wavelength, the second mode of resonance (Figure 3–3b) corresponds to ¾ of a wavelength, and the third mode (Figure 3–3c) corresponds to 5/4 of a wavelength. That is, there is a progression of modes whose wavelength increases in odd numbered multiples (1, 3, 5, . . .). This progression is an important characteristic of all tubes that are open at one end and closed at the other. A convenient summarizing tool is the equation shown in Figure 3–4.

This equation merely translates the above reasoning into a convenient summary device with which to calculate the resonant frequency of each mode. The equation also serves to delineate physical factors that can change the resonant frequency of a system. These factors are the mode number (k), the speed of sound in air (v), and the effective length (*L*). Features such as cross-sectional area and surface texture of the tube are not factors, and as such are not represented in the equation. These may affect the intensity of the resonance and damping characteristics, but not the frequency location of the resonance.

The expression (2k − 1) is a multiplier of odd numbers. If k = 1 (the first mode of resonance), then (2k − 1) is simply 1. If k =2 (the second mode of resonance), then (2k − 1) is 3. The first mode of the resonant frequency is therefore: $1 \times v/4L$. The second mode of resonance is $3 \times v/4L$, and so on with odd numbered multiples. (The speed of sound is usually taken to be 340,000 mm/sec or 340 m/sec.)

Examples of quarter wavelength resonators in musical instruments are the trumpet and the clarinet. These will be discussed in detail in Chapter 4. Figure 3–5 shows the resonant pattern of a clarinet playing the note concert F_5 (699 Hz) with the first mode of resonance at 699 Hz and the second at approximately 2100 Hz (three times the frequency of the first mode). Its third mode of resonance would be at 5 × 699 Hz, which is approximately 3500 Hz, and indeed, Figure 3–5 shows a small resonance at this frequency.

$F = (2k\text{-}1)\ v/4L$ where k is the mode number

v is the speed of sound

and *L* is the effective length

Figure 3–4. Equation for a quarter wavelength resonator. The primary factor affecting this type of resonance is the length of the tube (*L*).

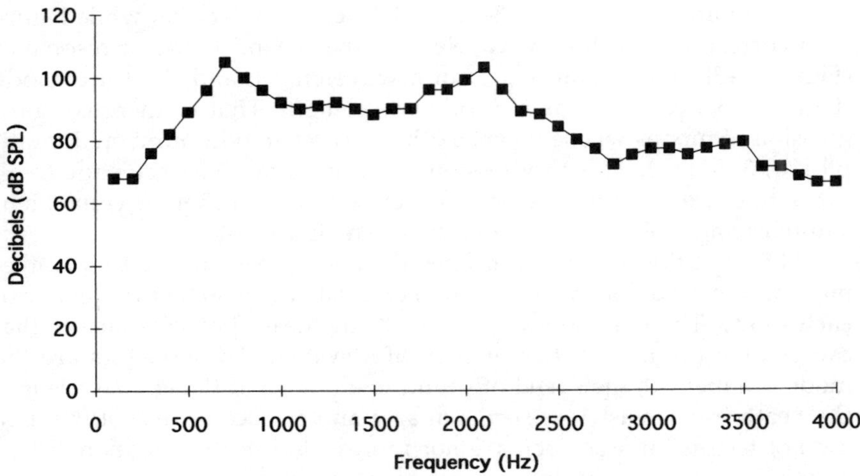

Figure 3–5. Resonant pattern (spectrum) of a clarinet playing concert F_5 (699 Hz). The clarinet functions as a quarter wavelength resonator—open at one end and closed at the other.

It should be pointed out that the effective length (*L*) is not always the measured length. We know from hearing aid acoustics that several factors can affect the calculation of effective length. These may include the effect of a bell or horn as well as unusual boundary conditions. Unusual boundary conditions with musical instruments may include the effect of the reed or mouthpiece. As in the case of hearing aid acoustics, the difference between actual length and effective length is relatively minor and is typically less than 5%. This difference is generally only observed for the lower frequencies for reasons given later in this chapter.

Half wavelength resonators also exist in the study of the acoustics of musical instruments. Oboes, bassoons, flutes, and violins are some examples. Unlike quarter wavelength resonators, half wavelength resonators have waveguides or tubes that are either open at both ends or closed at both ends. In the case of a violin, the strings are held tightly at both ends, at which point a node occurs (with an antinode in the middle of the string). In addition to the length, the resonant characteristics of stringed instruments are also related to the tension and the mass of the string. Figure 3–6 shows a tube that is closed at both ends and another that is open at both ends. Both of these tube boundary conditions will give rise to a similar pattern of resonances.

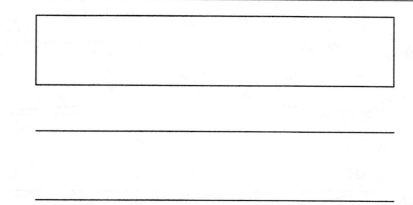

Figure 3–6. Two possible conditions for a one half wavelength resonator—open at both ends or closed at both ends.

The standing wave pattern for the first three modes of resonance are shown in Figures 3–7a, 3–7b, and 3–7c. Note that the first mode of this pattern indicates exactly one half of a wavelength—hence the name. It can be observed that the second mode of resonance is twice that of the first, and the third mode of resonance is three times that of the first mode. Thus, half wavelength resonators possess resonances that are integer multiples of the lowest frequency mode of resonance. Figure 3–8 shows the equation for the calculation of the set of resonant frequencies for a one half wavelength resonator.

Similar to the case for the quarter wavelength equation (in Figure 3–4), it is clear that the factors affecting the frequency location of the various modes of resonance are the speed of sound (which is relatively constant) and the effective length (*L*) of the resonator.

The second mode of resonance is always double the frequency of the first with this resonator type. Doubling of the frequency defines a one-octave increase. Therefore, for half wavelength resonators, such as the oboe and bassoon, an octave key is utilized that effectively doubles the frequency of the first mode. In contrast, quarter wavelength resonators such as the clarinet do not have octave keys. (These instruments have "register" keys that increase the note being played by a factor of three, or a twelfth.)

Figure 3–9 shows a spectrum for the flute (a one half wavelength resonator) for the note A_5 (880 Hz). The first mode of resonance can be seen at 880 Hz, with subsequent modes at 1760 Hz and at 2640 Hz.

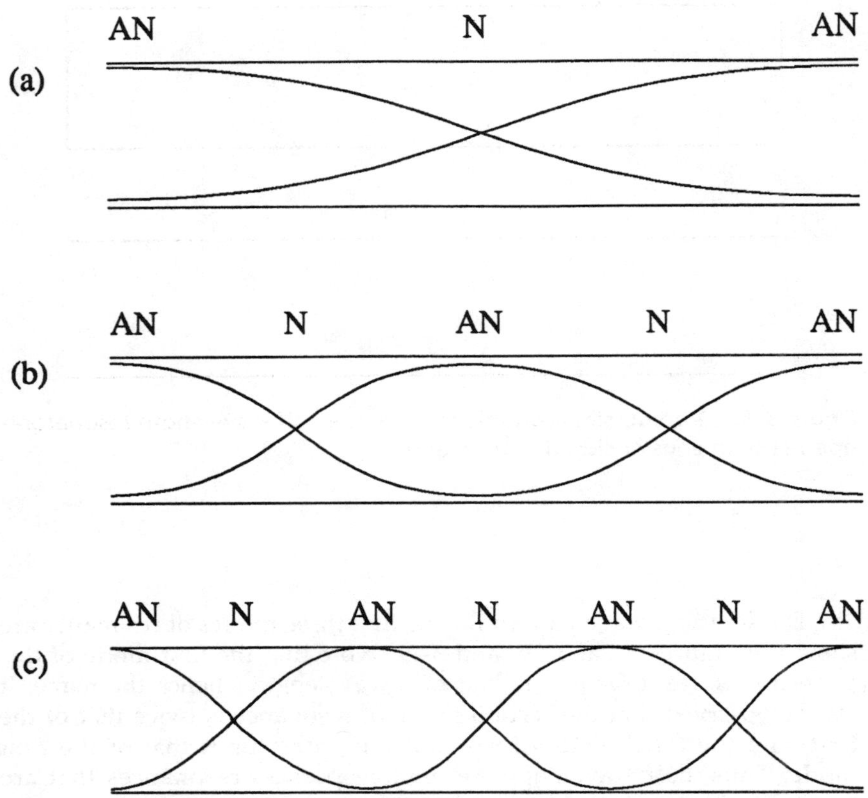

Figure 3–7. (a) First mode of resonance of a one half wavelength resonator (i.e., the lowest frequency resonance); (b) second mode of resonance of a one half wavelength resonator; (c) third mode of resonance of a one half wavelength resonator. N = node; AN = antinode.

Because of the exact nature of the boundary conditions, upper modes of resonance do not precisely follow the equations for quarter and half wavelength resonators. A full technical explanation for this deviant behavior is beyond the scope of this book, but the interested reader is referred to Benade (1990) or to Beranek (1986).

So far the discussion has revolved around tubes that are essentially cylindrical with no sudden changes in cross-sectional area. A sudden widening of a tube can create a discontinuity such that the wider tube can be thought of as a separate resonator with its own effective length. An example of a sudden widening can be found in a 2 cm long tube just

$F = k\,v/2L$ where k is the mode number
v is the speed of sound
and L is the effective length

Figure 3–8. Equation for a one half wavelength resonator. The primary factor affecting this type of resonance is the length of the tube (L).

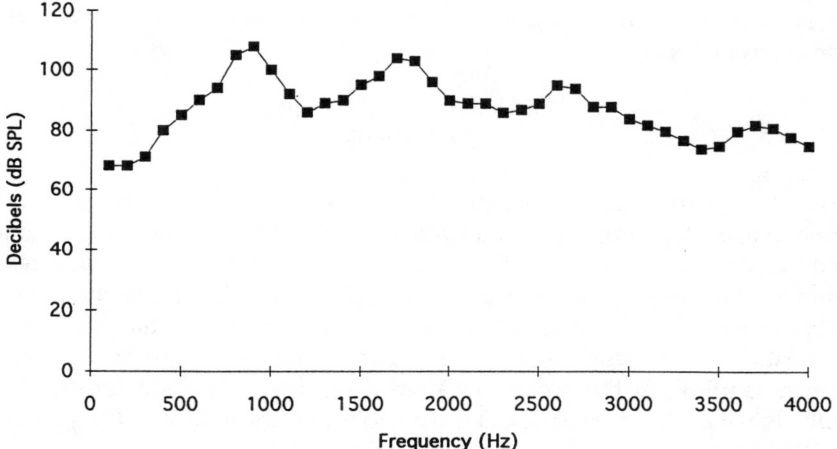

Figure 3–9. Resonant pattern (spectrum) of a flute playing A_5 (880 Hz). The flute functions as a one half wavelength resonator.

above the vocal chords of bass and baritone singers. Use of this resonating laryngeal tube (or expanded pharynx) has been shown to be useful in the creation of the "singer's formant" and is discussed in Chapter 4. Such an expanded pharynx is also of some linguistic use in many West African languages.

Mechanical and Helmholtz resonances are also found in the study of music. The violin possesses resonances relating to the volume of air enclosed in the body (referred to as *air resonances*) as well as mechanical resonances caused by the characteristics of the wood and its supporting structures (referred to as *wood resonances*). Virtually all instruments have resonances (or formants), which are an inherent side effect of their volume and shape. Tables 4–1, 4–2, and 4–3 (in Chapter 4) list many of the formants or resonances commonly found in musical instruments.

While wavelength resonances may be thought of as resonances within an element (such as a length of tubing), *Helmholtz resonances* may be thought of as resonances between elements. Specifically, a Helmholtz resonance is created by the interplay between a length of tubing (an acoustic mass) and an adjacent volume of air (an acoustic compliance). Blowing across the top of a pop bottle creates a Helmholtz resonance whose resonant frequency is defined by the length of the bottle neck and the volume of air in the bottle. The larger the volume of air, the lower will be the Helmholtz resonant frequency. Conversely, the greater the mass of air in the neck of the bottle, the higher will be the Helmholtz resonant frequency.

DAMPING

While resonance can be thought of as a selective amplification of certain frequencies depending on the characteristics of the system, *damping* may be thought of as attenuation of certain frequency regions. Unlike resonance, damping is not specific to certain calculable frequencies, but applies over a wide range of frequencies. The degree of damping of an acoustic system depends on the viscosity of air moving past a juncture (such as a hole at the bottom of a tympani), the wall characteristics in a tube (such as the interior of a clarinet tube), and the amount of impedance in the system (such as the presence of a mute or the diameter of a tube).

The degree of damping in a system defines the magnitude of the resonances. A system with a low amount of damping may have very high amplitude resonant peaks, whereas a highly damped system may have resonances that are barely discernable. Many loudspeakers are highly damped such that their frequency response appears to be "flat." It is not clear, however, that a highly damped system sounds better, but manufacturers of loudspeaker equipment tend to prefer the appearance of a flat frequency response curve.

The effects of damping may be observed when articulating a violin string. The placement of one's finger on a string will damp it slightly, relative to an open string. If one's goal is to determine the most intense sound that could be generated by a violin, it is therefore the best procedure to assess the sound level with an open string. Figure 3–10 shows two spectra: one of an open string on a violin and the other of the same note played on a lower string but articulated with the musician's finger. Note the increased damping (smaller magnitude resonant peaks) when the string is articulated.

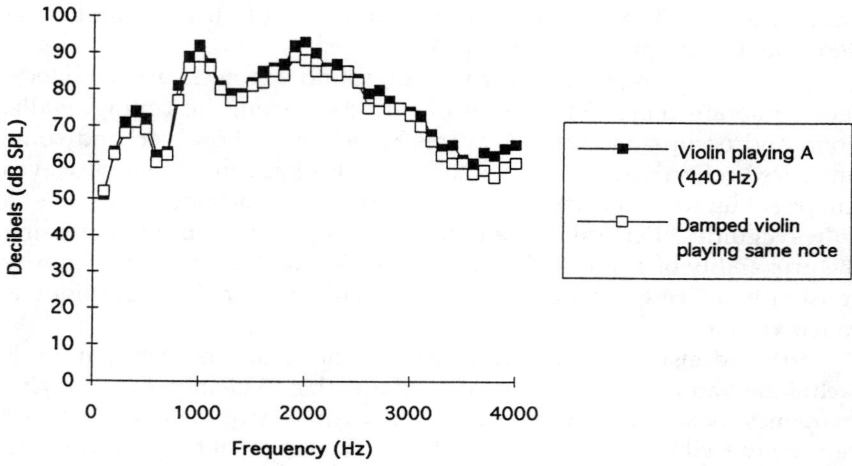

Figure 3–10. Two spectra of the same note on the violin A_4 (440 Hz), one being played on an open string, and the other being played on a lower string articulated with a finger.

Damping may also be observed as the hammer strikes a string in a piano. Playing an intense note will cause the felt covering of the hammer to compress, thus minimally damping the higher frequency components in the string. In contrast, playing the same note softly will cause a softer hammer head to damp out some of the higher frequency energy.

STANDING WAVES AND VIBRATO

Standing waves have been previously discussed in the study of resonance in tubes. They are the result of interference patterns set up by an incident wave interacting with a reflected wave moving in the opposite direction. Standing wave patterns can be observed in Figures 3–3 and 3–7.

Standing waves can also be set up in a performance venue. It is not uncommon, especially in a hall that was not designed to be acoustically optimal, for listeners to hear slightly different intensities of the music depending on the orientation of their head or exact seating position. In these cases, the incident music sound energy is interferring constructively and destructively with the reflected sound energy. It has been estimated that approximately 90% of the sound energy heard for speech is reflected energy, and there is no reason to assume that this is also not the case for music. Indeed, without this reflection, music would sound flat and empty. The optimal amount of reflection (which is frequency-dependent) is discussed in Chapter 7.

When designing a performance hall, sound engineers and architects seek to obtain the exact amount of reflection from the ceiling, walls, floor, and occupants. Rarely can this be achieved, however, and some undesired reflections are inevitable. When this happens, standing waves can be set up for some frequencies. That is, the performing venue acts as a "waveguide." Performers can ameliorate the situation by decreasing the probability of a reflected wave interferring with an incident wave by constantly altering the frequency by a small amount. This technique is called vibrato.

Stringed instrument players, such as violinists, consistently use this technique and at the professional level are able to change their playing frequency by about 6 Hz centered on the frequency of the note. Vocalists can create a vibrato of about 0.5% of their fundamental frequency, which corresponds to 1–2 Hz.

ACOUSTIC TRANSFORMER EFFECT

This effect forms the basis for the improvement in the transmission of high-frequency sounds. Specifically, the acoustic transformer effect enhances all frequencies whose one half wavelength is less than the total length of the tube. Mechanically this is accomplished by a gradual increase in the cross-sectional area of the tube (i.e., a horn). The discussion of the brass instruments in Chapter 4 indicates that the acoustic transformer effect enhances the intensity of every note that can be played.

Several general statements can be made about the acoustic behavior of flares or horns in musical instruments, and these derive from the mathematical modeling work of Daniel Bernoulli, Leonhard Euler, and Louis Lagrange in the mid-eighteenth century.

As a wave travels along a constantly flaring tube or waveguide, its pressure amplitude will gradually decrease because the wavefront is increasing. This is analogous to the gradual decrease in intensity of a flashlight beam as the distance from the flashlight is increased. Eventually the pressure disturbance will be adjacent to a region with a relatively low-pressure amplitude—namely the external environment at the end of the bell or flare of the musical instrument. If there is a significant mismatch in the pressure amplitude and associated impedance, much of the pressure disturbance will be reflected back to the source. Such a reflection contributes to the standing wave interference pattern set up in the musical instrument. A bell or flare is designed to improve this impedance mismatch, thus improving the transmission of sound, especially for the higher frequencies.

A sudden flaring of the musical instrument tubing (such as that found in the trumpet, French horn, and trombone), causes an increase in the velocity of sound with the low frequencies being reflected back to the source earlier than the higher frequency sounds. Subsequently, the suddenly flaring horn causes the lower frequency resonances to be shifted to a slightly higher frequency (shorter effective length) with no significant shift for the higher frequency components. This same phenomenon is observed in hearing aid earmold acoustics, where an earmold horn shifts the first three resonances up (to about 3500 Hz) in frequency slightly but leaves the fourth and fifth resonant locations intact.

In contrast, for those instruments possessing a gradual flaring (such as the baritone and fluegel horn), there will be no shift in the frequency of the lower resonances, even though the flare will still serve to enhance the transmission of the higher frequencies. Chapter 4 delineates some of the beneficial attributes for this lack of shift for these instruments.

A mute that is ocassionally used with a trumpet (which has the effect of undoing much of the acoustic transformer effect) will not only decrease the high-frequency transmission of sound, but will also shift the lower frequency resonances down in frequency.

A third general characteristic of a flare or horn (in a brass instrument) is that the lower frequency sound components spread out around the bell evenly in all directions, whereas higher frequency components tend to be oriented in a line along the playing axis of the instrument. This high-frequency directional characteristic for belled brass instruments is discussed further in Chapter 4 and forms the basis for why trumpets should be on risers (see Chapter 8). For the vowel [a] (as in "f<u>a</u>ther"), the acoustic transformer effect enhances the intensity for all sounds over 1500 Hz. Opening one's mouth to its fullest position essentially allows for an optimal transmission for the higher frequency formants and higher frequency harmonics.

Figure 3–11 shows the improvement in the transmission of the higher frequency components when the vowel [a] is articulated with the mouth held wide open as compared with the mouth in a relaxed position.

Thomas Edison understood the acoustic transformer effect and used it as a volume control on his early Victorola record players. The playback needle was coupled with a flare or horn that was approximately 1000 millimeters in length. This horn enhanced the sound transmission for all frequencies above 170 Hz (i.e., $340{,}000/[2 \times 1000] = 170$ Hz), which effectively increased the sound intensity for all the sounds that were transduced. A tennis ball-sized baffle connected to a cable was utilized in the horn as a damping agent. As the cable was retracted (by the listener adjusting the "volume" control) the ball was drawn closer to the narrow neck of the horn, thus reducing the acoustic transformer effect.

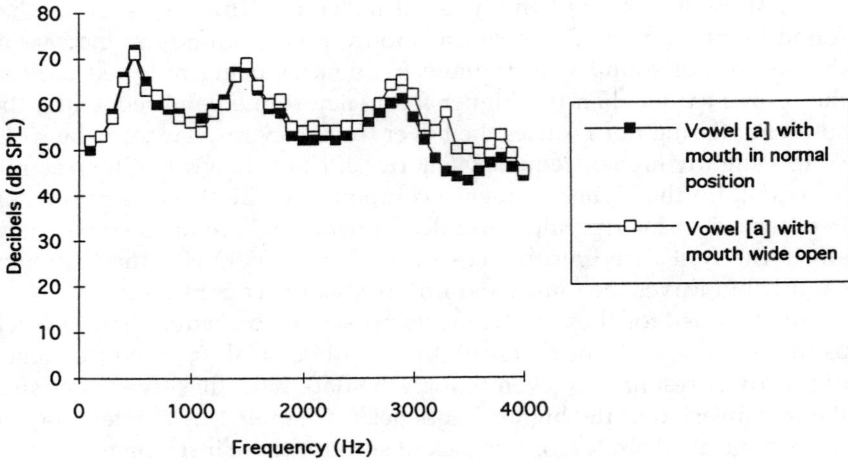

Figure 3–11. Two spectra of the vowel [a] for the mouth in a relaxed position, and held wide open.

HIGH-FREQUENCY REFLECTIVITY AND IMPEDANCE

Closely related to the acoustic transformer effect, higher frequency sounds tend to reflect. A technical description of this principle is that the acoustic impedance of the acoustic inertance is proportional to frequency. An "English translation" is that high frequencies don't like small spaces. Much of the behavior of this acoustic principle is related to the wavelength of the sound.

Sound waves tend to be "visually myopic" in the sense that a different impedance or blockage is seen by an obstruction depending on the frequency. The degree of acoustic reflection is proportional to frequency. Low-frequency sound energy possesses long wavelengths and do not "see" many obstructions as being acoustically significant. Low frequencies are transmitted through obstructions such as walls and people without much attenuation or reflection. In contrast, much of the higher frequency energy tends to be reflected by an obstruction.

Specifically, sound energy will be obstructed and reflected to the source if one half of its wavelength approaches the diameter of the obstruction. The body baffle and head shadow effects are well-known examples of this, where the human body and head may cause an attenuation of the higher frequency sound energy. For example, a head that is 20 cm in diameter (between the ears) obstructs frequencies that have one half wavelengths shorter than 20 cm.

This corresponds to 850 Hz. Sound energy below 850 Hz, therefore, does not view the head as an obstruction, whereas higher frequency sounds are increasingly obstructed. In essence, there is an acoustic shadow created for the higher frequencies on the nonsignal side of the head. The head shadow effect is one of the rationales provided for the benefits of binaural (two sided) amplification.

As will be discussed in Chapter 7, performance halls may have an undesirable level of high-frequency reflection, referred to as reverberation. A person in the lobby of the performance hall of a rock concert or a Broadway musical will tend to hear the low-frequency sounds relatively unaffected but will miss out the higher frequency components. This effect will also be discussed in Chapter 5 and is crucial to the understanding of why ear protection (unless specifically designed) will attenuate the higher frequency sounds more than the lower frequency ones. As a result, most of these high-frequency sounds either are absorbed by the walls and content of the room or are reflected into the theatre or performance hall, contributing to the reverberation.

SOUND DIRECTIVITY

As stated above, the degree of acoustic reflection is proportional to frequency. Inside the bell of a trumpet, short wavelength (i.e., high-frequency) sounds acoustically see the wall of the instrument as an obstruction and therefore view it as a waveguide. In contrast, lower frequency sound energy (being acoustically myopic) does not see the trumpet wall as much of a waveguide and tends to spread out in all directions about the trumpet player. For low-frequency sounds, a sound level meter placed at 45° above the playing plane of the trumpet will record a similar level as if it were placed in the playing plane. In contrast, for higher frequency sounds, the trumpet is highly directional. Figure 3–12 shows this characteristic for a trumpet where the measuring angles above (+45°) and below (−45°) the playing plane of the trumpet are compared with low-, mid-, and high-frequency sounds.

Speaker systems also have directional characteristics. Speakers with open-backed cabinets can radiate as much sound from their uncovered rear than from the front (especially for the lower frequencies where the depth of the enclosure approaches one quarter of a wavelength) and undesirable enhancements and cancellations of sounds may be achieved due to phase interactions.

Even closed-backed speakers have directional characteristics and these are based on the vibration patterns of the various speaker cones. Typically, the tweeters that transduce the higher frequencies emit sounds in a tighter beam than the larger woofers. Elevating speakers

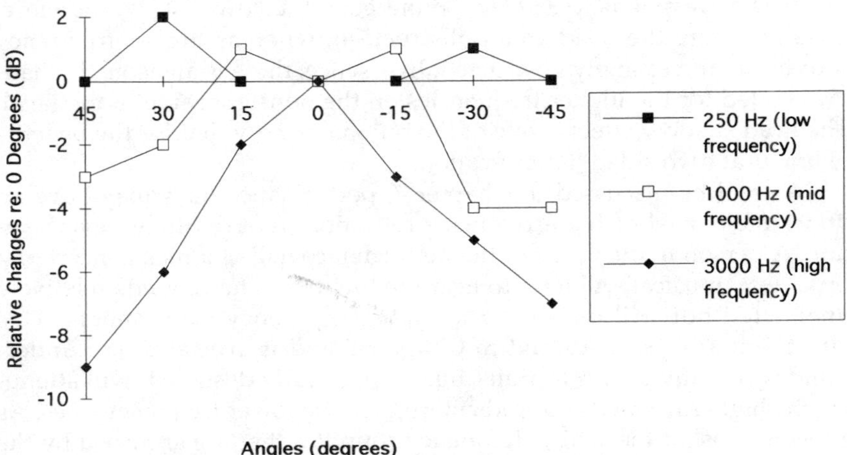

Figure 3–12. The relative output of a trumpet as measured above (positive angles) and below (negative angles) the playing plane.

that transduce significant high-frequency energy would allow much of this potentially damaging source of music exposure to literally go over the heads of many musicians.

It is commonplace to assess a musician clinically who has recently moved from one city to another but is employed by the same popular music show, and find that one performance pit is significantly worse than another. More often than not, the better performance pit had its speakers elevated relative to that of the worse venue.

Beranek (1986) provides an excellent technical expansion of this topic for the interested reader. The directional characteristics of some musical instruments will be found in Chapter 4.

SUMMARY

A technical basis has been provided for the understanding of subsequent chapters of this book (specifically, musical instruments, hearing protectors, and environmental modifications).

Quarter and half wavelength resonators were introduced that form the basis for the physics of musical instruments and vocalists. Examples of quarter wavelength resonators are the trumpet and the clarinet. Examples of half wavelength resonators are oboes, bassoons, flutes, and violins. In addition, Helmholtz and mechanical resonances are also of importance. These resonances may be related to an enclosed volume of air, or the characteristics of the instrument materials.

Damping reduces the magnitude of the resonances and may be related to the presence of felt on a piano hammer, or even one's finger touching a violin string.

The physics of bells or flares is associated with an enhancement of higher frequency sound energy, and depending on the length of the bell, the entire spectrum of that instrument may be amplified.

High frequencies don't like small spaces. The physics of this statement underscores the importance of baffles and reflecting shields used in many music performance halls.

A related concept is sound directivity where high-frequency sounds are more directional than lower frequency sounds. Ramifications of this concept can be found in loudspeaker placement and, as will be discussed in subsequent chapters, the use of risers for trumpet players.

CHAPTER

4

The Physics of Musical Instruments

INTRODUCTION

This chapter will equip the audiologist with information to answer some basic questions regarding the acoustics of a wide range of musical instruments. No previous knowledge of music is required but there are many similarities between the physics discussed here and that of the human voice as well as in hearing aid acoustics. There are some excellent reference books on this area to which the interested reader is referred. From a lay approach, increasing to a technical mathematical approach, the reader is referred to Backus (1977), Campbell and Greated (1987), Benade (1990), Roederer (1995), and Fletcher and Rossing (1991).

This chapter provides an overview of the relevant acoustic characteristics of six classes of musical instruments and the human voice. All of the physical phenomena and acoustic principles were covered previously in Chapter 3. As will be observed, some of the measured acoustic phenomena of musical instruments are inherent in the design, some are related to a conscious manipulation of resonances (formants), and some are related to the playing technique of the various musicians. The assessment paradigm discussed in Chapter 6 will allow for the generation of acoustic spectra of various instruments, but the bases of the expected acoustic behavior are discussed here. Most of the spectra in this chapter have been generated with the technique discussed in Chapter 6.

The seven classes of instruments (with examples) are:

1. piano (piano and harpsichord)
2. woodwinds (clarinet, saxophone, oboe, bassoon)
3. flute (flute, picollo)
4. brass (trumpet, trombone, French horn)
5. strings (violin, viola, cello, bass)
6. percussion (gongs, bar, glockenspiel, tympani)
7. the human voice.

While there are other instruments, the vast majority is covered. In cases where a specific instrument is not covered, it will generally fit into one of the seven categories mentioned above.

An instrument may have a certain measured spectrum if a musician plays it at one level, and quite a differently shaped spectrum for the identical note if played at a different level. Whenever possible, the explanations for these differences will be discussed. This is typically the case for the piano and woodwinds. Spectra for the other classes of instruments maintain their respective shapes regardless of the playing intensity—altered only by a shifting up or down of the entire spectrum in intensity as the playing level is varied. A question such as "What is a typical spectrum of a certain instrument?" may be meaningless if reference is not made to playing level for the piano and woodwinds.

For some instruments the measured acoustic spectra may be relatively unimportant for the proper perception. That is, analogous to the study of linguistic phonology, there is a "phonetic spectrum" and a "phonemic spectrum." The *phonetic spectrum* is the actual measured output of an instrument. The *phonemic spectrum* is the set of cues relevent for a particular class of musicians. For example, despite the fact that a violin and a clarinet may have similar high-frequency energy components in their (phonetic) spectrum, a clarinet player is not required to hear the higher frequency components for a good sound. In contrast, it is crucial for a violinist to be aware of the magnitude of the higher frequency harmonics. Thus one may say that despite an apparent similarity between the spectra of violins and clarinets, the phonemic spectra (or perceptive requirements) differ radically, with the violin spectrum having much more importance in the higher frequency regions.

An analysis of these differences leads to some important strategies for reducing the potential for hearing loss among various musician groups. These strategies and approaches will be discussed throughout this book. Whereas the properties of the phonetic spectrum can be ascertained from knowledge of the physics of acoustics as well as by a direct spectral assessement, the phonemic spectra comes from interviewing over one thousand musicians of various instrument classes and playing styles over a number of years. Phonemic spectra are therefore less exact than phonetic ones, but the general properties are well understood and will be presented here whenever possible.

SOURCE–FORMANT FILTER–RADIATION MODEL

A convenient model (shown in Figure 4–1a with an example in Figure 4–1b) that summarizes many of the acoustic properties of musical instruments is the Source–Formant Filter–Radiation model. This is similar to that used in the study of the output of the human vocal tract.

The *source* has energy at a fundamental frequency and higher frequency harmonics and overtones. *Harmonics* are components that bear an integer relationship to the fundamental frequency and *overtones* are those that do not necessarily coincide with an integer multiple of the fundamental frequency. Examples of a source may be the vocal chords, bow and strings, reed(s), and other vibrating structures such as the lips in brass instruments.

These sources of vibration serve as an input to the musical instrument, which in turn have resonances (or formants) that are either inherent (such as the enclosed air in a violin or a resonance of a soundboard) or specific to the note being played (such as the length of available tubing in a trombone). These formants function as a filter by altering the amplitude of the fundamental and harmonics of the source. Like the analogous model of the vocal tract, these formants are independent of the source vibrations. Unless specifically intended (e.g., formant tuning for soprano singers), there is no reason to assume that a harmonic will be at a formant frequency other than by coincidence. As observed in Figure 4–1b, the harmonics in a formant region, however, will be enhanced in magnitude.

Finally, depending on the physical construction of the instrument, sound radiates to the environment, which depends intimately on what physicists call *boundary conditions.* Examples of boundary conditions are the flare or bell at the end of brass instruments or the vocal tract, the orientation and location of f-holes in a stringed instrument, and even the geometry of finger holes in a woodwind instrument.

In the following discussion, reference will be made to these three aspects pertaining to the acoustic output of the instruments. Whenever possible, resonances or formants will be delineated (see Tables 4–1, 4–2, 4–3, further in the chapter) so that they will be recognized in the phonetic spectrum of the instrument being assessed in Chapter 6.

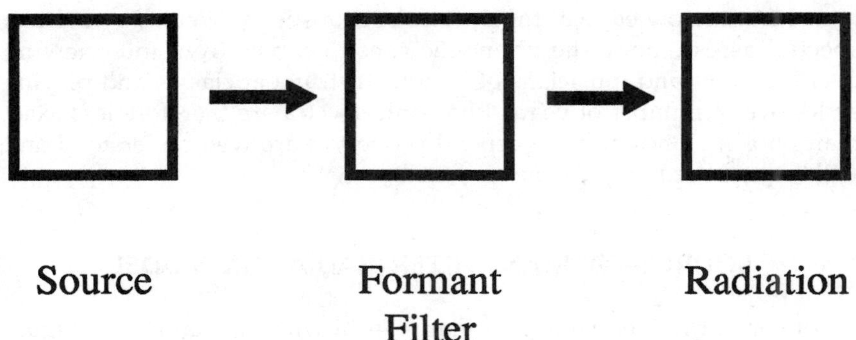

Figure 4–1a. A model of three independent aspects of sound production: the sound source, the formant filter, and the radiation characteristics.

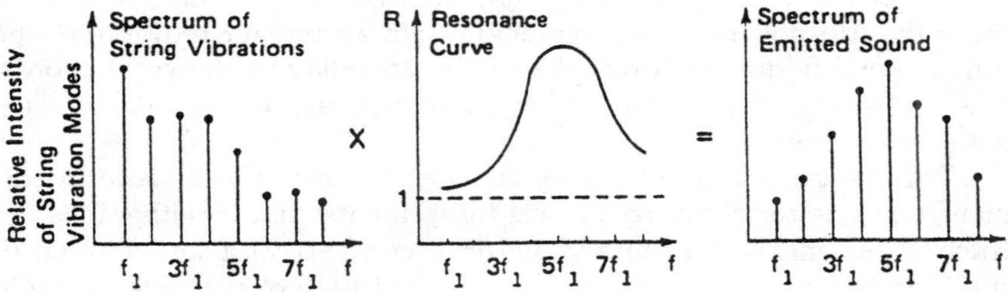

Figure 4–1b. Source spectrum combined with a formant pattern, yielding an output spectrum. (From *The Physics and Psychophysics of Music* [p. 128], by J. G. Roederer, 1995, New York: Springer-Verlag. Copyright 1995 by Springer-Verlag New York, Inc. Reprinted with permission.)

For consistency, the note-to-frequency nomenclature has been chosen according to the octaves on a piano keyboard starting with the lowest note A_0 (27.5 Hz). Beginning with each C a new subscript is used denoting successive octaves. Middle C is then C_4 (262 Hz) and the top note on the piano keyboard is C_8 (4186 Hz). Other systems are in use today and they are equally valid. The frequency (in Hz) will generally be appended to the note in question. A full conversion chart of musical note-to-frequency is found in Appendix I.

INSTRUMENT CLASSES

Piano

The piano was invented in 1709 as a modification of the harpsichord, which allowed musical notes to be played over a range of intensities, from a very soft (pianissimo), to a very loud (fortissimo) level. The original name was therefore the pianoforte, which has been shortened to, simply, the piano. This instrument has a series of strings of pre-set length that are clamped tightly at both ends (between the capo d'astro bar and the hitch pin). The bridge sits directly on the soundboard and vibrations are transduced directly from the strings to the soundboard. Reinforcing ribs are designed to run across the grain of the soundboard to provide a certain impedance and associated sound intensity. The impedance of the soundboard can be affected by the wood thickness, rib density, wood quality (graininess), type, and number of ribs. Depending on these factors, various pianos will have slightly different formants that serve to enhance different frequencies. Unlike most other instruments, the formant structure of pianos can vary widely and is a major reason why one piano sounds better than another.

The strings function primarily as a one half wavelength resonator (see Chapter 3) with a length extending from the capo d'astro bar to the bridge of the piano. Because the bridge is elastically coupled to the soundboard, which moves slightly, the effective length of the vibrating string is somewhat longer and the higher frequency energy components are not always at integer multiples of the fundamental. In addition, long strings tend to have a slight inharmonicity associated with them so, in order to minimize this problem, they need to be stretched very tightly—almost to the breaking point. Strings stretched this tightly have a high impedence and an associated low playing intensity. For this reason, each piano note is made up of several strings.

Another major feature of the piano that affects the acoustic output is the nature of the felt on the hammers, which strike the strings. If the felt is soft, or equivalently, if the hammer strikes the strings without much force (as in pianissimo), there will be some damping of the higher frequency components. In contrast, if the felt is hard, or equivalently, if the hammer strikes the strings with great force (as in fortissimo), there is compression of the felt with minimal damping of the higher frequency components. When the note being played is fortissimo, there will subsequently be a greater dynamic range in the higher frequencies than if hit with a pianissimo force. Figure 4–2 shows such a comparison with the same note [A_4 (440 Hz)] being played at both a pianissimo and a fortissimo level. Questions pertaining to the exact spectral shape of a note on the piano are meaningless unless the playing level is specified.

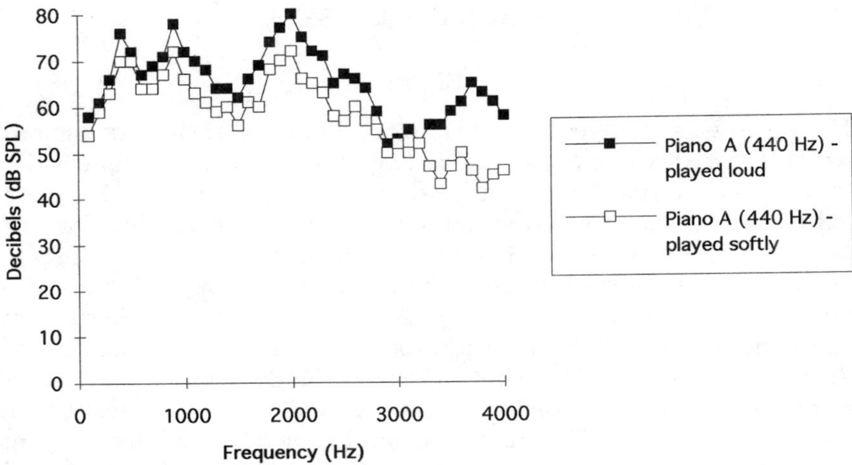

Figure 4–2. A comparison of the piano playing A_4 (440 Hz) at a pianissimo and a fortissimo playing level.

A final element that may affect the acoustic output of a piano is the angle of the lid on a grand piano. The volume of trapped air as well as the reflective characteristics of the piano top will serve to alter the piano's output spectrum.

Clearly, these acoustic factors, which may vary significantly from piano to piano, do not affect electronically amplified pianos or keyboards. There is no inherent electronic reason that there should be any difference in high-frequency sound transmission as a function of playing level, other than if instrument design engineers intentionally choose to implement this feature.

The notes on a full-sized piano keyboard span more than seven octaves and range from A_0 (27.5 Hz) to C_8 (4186 Hz). The playing intensity varies with pianist, style, and instrument but typically ranges from 40 dB SPL for the softest sound (ppp) to 110 dB SPL for the most intense sound (fff).

Harpsichords are undergoing a resurgence in popularity. These precursors to the piano differ in three essential acoustic ways:

1. no hammer-induced volume control
2. thinner strings than a piano with an associated lower intensity level
3. an enclosed air cavity below the soundboard that provides additional formants.

The sound level emanating from a harsichord is therefore lower than that of a piano, with virtually no dynamic range. The formant structure caused by the soundboard as well as the air cavity below the soundboard is different from that of a piano.

Reeded Woodwinds

These instruments include the clarinet, saxophone, oboe, bassoon, and English horn. The flute deserves a separate section because of its lack of a reed. Unlike most other musical instruments, the clarinet and saxophone are tuned two semitones lower and are termed B-flat instruments (rather than C). When clarinet players are asked to play concert C, they will need to play B flat in order to be in tune with the rest of the orchestra (i.e., concert pitch). This alternative tuning was designed to slightly increase the range of these instruments.

The source element for these instruments is of course the reed and it functions by an interplay between the resting position of the reed on the mouthpiece and the Bernoulli principle (see Chapter 3). The Bernoulli principle states that pressure is inversely related to the velocity of air. As a musician blows into the mouthpiece, the high velocity of air passing the reed creates a low pressure zone, thus causing the reed to move toward the mouthpiece facing. As it does, the airflow is gradually reduced, with a subsequent returning of the reed to its rest position. The reed typically undergoes complete closure with the mouth piece facing only for those notes played louder than a mezzo forte level.

The woodwinds can be divided into two subclasses based on acoustic resonance. The first class of woodwinds uses single reeds (usually manufactured in France from a type of cane called Arundo Donax). The clarinet and the saxophone are members of this class and function as quarter wavelength resonators (similar to the acoustics of ear molds in hearing aids) because of their essentially cylindrical shape that is "closed" at the reed end and "open" at the "other end." The other end is at the first open hole. That is, as the finger holes are opened in a clarinet, the cylinder is effectively shortened, with an increase in the frequency of the note being played. Figure 4–3 shows a stylized clarinet with open circles marking the open holes. The note shown in this figure is middle C [which is concert D_4 (294 Hz)] and the acoustic length is denoted by *L*. The remainder of the clarinet (or saxophone) barrel below this point is acoustically irrelevant; detaching the bottom portion of this instrument has minimal effect.

Since quarter wavelength resonators have resonances or formants at odd number multiples of the first mode (see Chapter 3), overblowing the clarinet or saxophone will result in a resonant frequency that is three times that of the first mode. An octave would be double the first mode

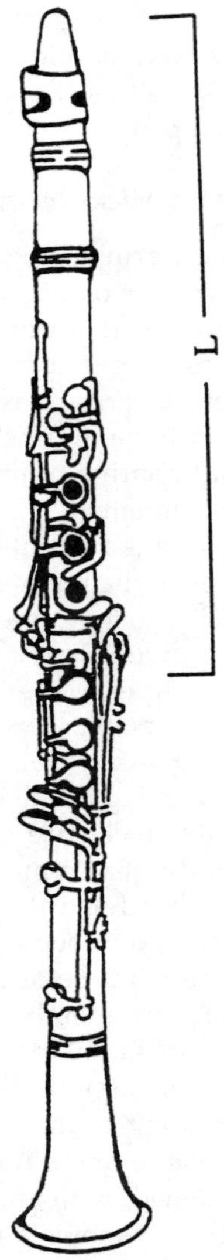

Figure 4–3. A stylized clarinet with the open circles indicating the noncovered finger holes. The acoustic length (*L*) extends to the first noncovered finger hole.

[i.e., C_4 (262 Hz) to C_5 (524 Hz)], but with clarinets and saxophones, overblowing would result in C_4 (262 Hz) to G_5 (784 Hz)—a full octave and one fifth (or a twelfth). This is why clarinets and saxophones have "register" keys and not octave keys. Figure 4–4 shows two spectra of a clarinet for concert G_5 [i.e., F_5 (699 Hz)] played at both a mezzo forte and a forte level. Note the increase in the higher frequencies for the forte level note relative to that of the quieter mezzo forte level.

The second class of woodwinds is conical in shape—steadily increasing in cross-sectional area from the reed end to the open end of the instrument. Conical acoustics tend to be more complicated than that for the cylinder, but these instruments (oboe, basoon, and English horns) function primarily as one half wavelength resonators (with secondary quarter-wavelength characteristics). Overblowing these instruments will result in an octave increase because half wavelength resonators have modes of resonance that are integer multiples of the first mode. A double reed is utilized for these instruments.

Reeds always lower the frequency of the resonances in the air column and the stiffer the reed, the higher will be the resonant frequency. Most beginners start with a low-strength reed (2 or 2½), whereas more accomplished musicians tend to use a higher strength reed (3 or 4). The higher the strength of the reed, the greater will be the high-frequency sound energy transmission. For high-strength reeds, there is a playing intensity/high-frequency interaction similar to that found with the piano and a hard felt covering for the hammer. Note that there is virtually no intensity increase for the fundamental energy for the two playing levels in Figure 4–4.

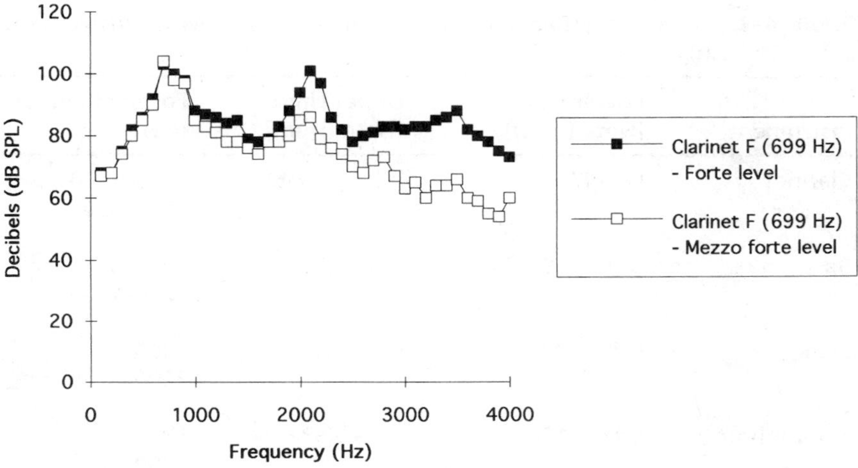

Figure 4–4. Two spectra of a clarinet playing concert G_5 [i.e., F_5 (699 Hz)], played at both a mezzo forte level and a forte level.

This high-frequency "playing intensity" cue is found for all woodwinds. Perhaps the only important aspect of the high- frequency part of the spectrum for reeded woodwinds is this intensity cue. Despite the existance of this cue, experienced woodwind players tend to rely on their sensation of air pressure build-up behind the reed as their playing intensity cue. For these musicians, the phonemic spectrum would have little high-frequency importance. As will be discussed in Chapter 5, dependence on this high-frequency cue may necessitate an alternate form of ear protection. Reeded woodwind players rely on the low-frequency interresonant breathiness or noise as their indication of a good tone. Dependence on the upper harmonics contributes little to the sense of playing.

The frequency ranges of some woodwind instruments are shown in Table 4–1 (concert pitch) along with formants that are an inherent result of their dimensions and shape.

A final point about reeded woodwinds concerns the radiation of the sound to the environment. For low- and mid-frequency sounds, reeded woodwinds are nondirectional; however, for the higher frequency sounds they become more directional along the playing axis of the instrument. That is, for high-frequency notes, the main sound energy comes out along the direction of the bell and is not heard by the musician as well as lower frequency notes. Depending on the performing environment (see Chapter 7), this high-frequency energy may or may

Table 4–1. Frequency Ranges and Formants of Woodwind Instruments (Concert Pitch)

Instrument	Lower Limit [Note (freq)]	Upper Limit [Note (freq)]	Formant Regions (Hz)
Clarinet	D_3(147)	B $flat_6$(1865)	1500–1700 3700–4300
Bassoon	B $flat_1$(58)	E $flat_5$(622)	440–500 1200–1300
Oboe	B $flat_3$(233)	F_6(1397)	1400 3000
English horn	E $flat_3$(156)	B $flat_5$(932)	930 2300
Flute	C_4(262)	C_7(2093)	800

not be heard by the audience. For a musical note assessment, Benade (1990) suggests placing a microphone at the opening of the first open hole. Although this will provide a valid spectrum for that one note, it is understandably not a reasonable approach for a live performance. For this reason, recording reeded woodwind instruments is very difficult and rarely can there be a true duplication of the sound.

Flute

Although modern day flutes are rarely made of wood, they nevertheless are still considered woodwind instruments. The modern day flute (that is 670 mm long) consists of three sections: the head joint, which contains the mouth hole and can be used for tuning, the main body joint, incorporating most of the keys that cover air holes, and the foot joint, which incorporates the key for the baby finger on the right hand. The piccolo is physically half as long as the flute and is subsequently one octave higher.

The musician blows across the opening of the flute mouth hole, creating a flow-controlled valve. Helmholtz worked out the basic principles and they are summarized here. When a musician blows across the opening of the mouth hole, some air flows into the opening. Depending on the resonance of the flute (or bottle), there is a subsequent outflow of air, which serves to deflect the musician's breath outward. When the outflow is complete, the breath is again oriented across the opening of the air hole. This cycle continues at a rate in accordance with the resonant frequency of the flute or bottle. The lips of the musician do not oscillate as they do with brass musicians.

Like reeded woodwinds, the resonant frequency is defined by the volume up to the first noncovered air hole. It is at this location that the sound radiates from the instrument.

When a musician's breath (airstream) is used to maintain a vibration in the flute, the airstream itself can alter the resonance. If the musician blows softly, the note tends to be flat, and if blown hard, the note tend to be sharp. It is not unusual to hear a flutist play a crescendo (getting louder) and a decrecendo (getting softer) sharp and then flat.

As can be seen in Table 4–1, the flute ranges from a low note of C_4 (262 Hz) to a high note of C_7 (2093 Hz) with a formant at 800 Hz. A formant in the 800 Hz region means that the note G_5 will be enhanced in intensity regardless of the playing level. Figure 4–5 shows a spectrum for the flute of A_5 (880 Hz). The fundamental of A_5 (880 Hz) is near the flute's formant at 800 Hz, which serves to enhance the intensity of this note. Since the flute is a one half wavelength resonantor, one would expect its second harmonic to be one octave higher (at 1760 Hz) and indeed this is clearly observed in Figure 4–5.

Unlike most other musicians, symmetrical hearing is crucial for most flute players. It is not unusual for flutists to complain of distortion

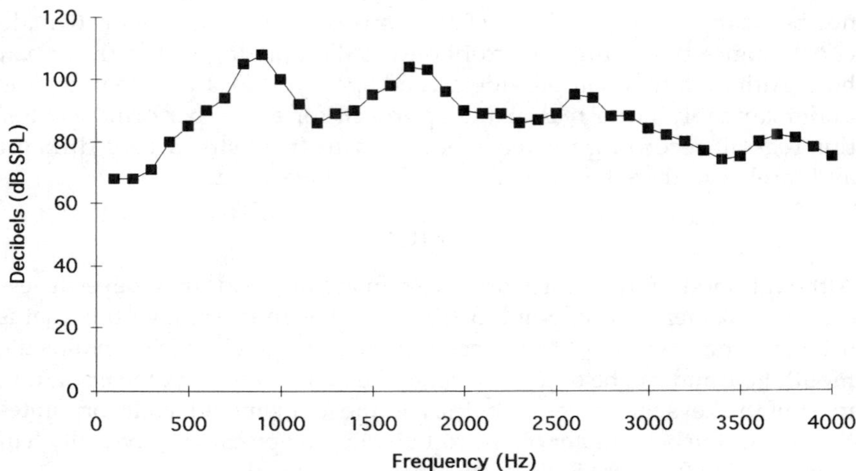

Figure 4–5. A spectrum of a flute playing A_5 (880 Hz). This note is near the formant frequency of the flute (at 800 Hz) that serves to enhance its intensity. The note A_5 (880 Hz) cannot be played at a pianissimo level.

in their better ear. Because of the orientation of the flute to the right hand side, the left ear is less prone to a music-induced hearing loss. The ability of the left ear to pick up high-frequency harmonics that are not heard in the poorer right ear may be perceived as undesirable distortion. A fitting of asymmetrical vented/tuned earplugs (as discussed in Chapter 5) that yields balanced high-frequency hearing at the eardrum is a very useful tool for these musicians.

Brass

Brass instruments have three sections: the mouthpiece, a variable length of tubing, and a bell. Figure 4–6 shows a stylized brass instrument. The length can be altered by the use of valves or by the introduction of additional tubing.

Brass instruments are the only ones that do not adhere to the Source–Formant Filter–Radiation model shown in Figure 4–1a. The vibrations at the musician's lips are not independent of the mechanical characteristics of the instrument "downstream." Lip vibration depends on the acoustic pressure developed in the mouthpiece, as well as by feedback effects of the instrument tubing. For a detailed analysis of the interaction effects of lip vibration and brass instruments, the reader is referred to Benade (1973) for a nontechnical analysis or to Ayers (1995) for a mathematical description.

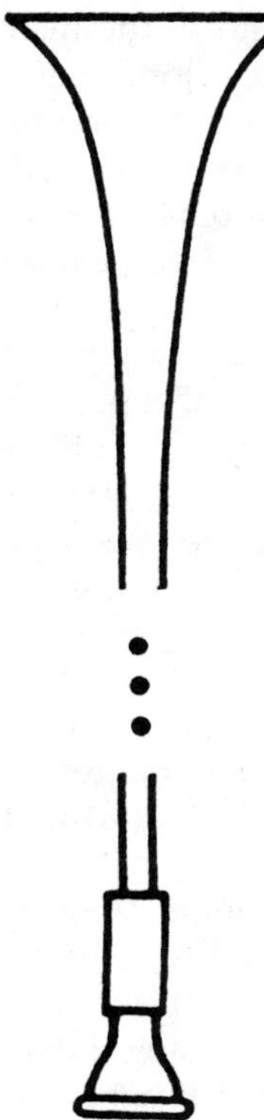

Figure 4–6. A stylized brass instrument showing the mouthpiece, the bell, and a variable length of tubing that can be altered with valves, or a slide.

Brass instruments function essentially like a quarter wavelength resonator that is closed at the mouthpiece and open near the end of the bell. The effective length is not only affected by the actual tubing length, but by the nature of the bell.

Like the reeded woodwinds, brass instruments can be divided into two groups based on the acoustic properties of the bell or horn. The first class of brass instruments has flaring horns and include the trumpet, the trombone, and the French horn. With a flaring horn, the sound pressure wave gradually increases in velocity as it approaches the open end. The acoustic result is that the effective length of the instrument is less than the measured length, with a higher set of resonant frequencies relative to a nonflaring instrument of identical physical length.

In contrast, the second class of brass instruments utilizes a cone rather than a flare. A cone has a constant increase in cross-sectional area from the mouthpiece to the end of the instrument. The associated resonances are at a lower frequency (longer effective length than an equivalent flared instrument) and would be more appropriate for bass instruments. Examples of brass instruments with cones are the baritone and the fluegel horn. Because cone brass instruments have lower magnitude high-frequency resonances, special mouthpieces are necessary to enhance the higher frequencies.

All brass instruments have a bell, regardless of its exact shape. The acoustic transformer effect (see Chapter 3) enhances those frequencies whose one half wavelength is less than the length of the tubing and bell. For a trumpet with a physical length of 1840 mm, the bell would enhance the intensity of all frequencies above 93 Hz, which corresponds to all notes above G_2 (98 Hz). Since the lowest note on a trumpet is E_3 (165 Hz), the bell serves to enhance every note that can be played by the trumpet. This reasoning extends to all brass instruments and explains why bass brass instruments must have longer tubing than the treble brass instruments. The frequency ranges of some brass instruments are shown in Table 4–2 along with the formants that are an inherent result of their dimensions and shape.

Unlike woodwind instruments, the sound radiates from the end of the bell. Mutes can then be used to reduce the output, especially for the higher frequencies by counteracting the bell-induced acoustic transformer action as well as by increasing the overall damping of the system.

Like reeded woodwind instruments, the radiation characteristics of brass instruments are highly directional but only for the higher frequencies. Figure 4–7 shows the directional characteristics of a trumpet if measured on the playing plane of the trumpet and if measured at 45° below the playing plane. Placing the trumpet section on risers will therefore serve to prevent much of the damaging high-frequency sound energy

Table 4–2. Frequency Ranges and Formants of Brass Instruments (Concert Pitch)

Instrument	Lower Limit [Note (freq)]	Upper Limit [Note (freq)]	Formant Regions (Hz)
Trumpet	E_3(165)	B flat$_5$(932)	1200–1400 2500
Trombone	E_2(82)	B flat$_4$(466)	600–800
French horn	B_1(62)	F_5(698)	400–500

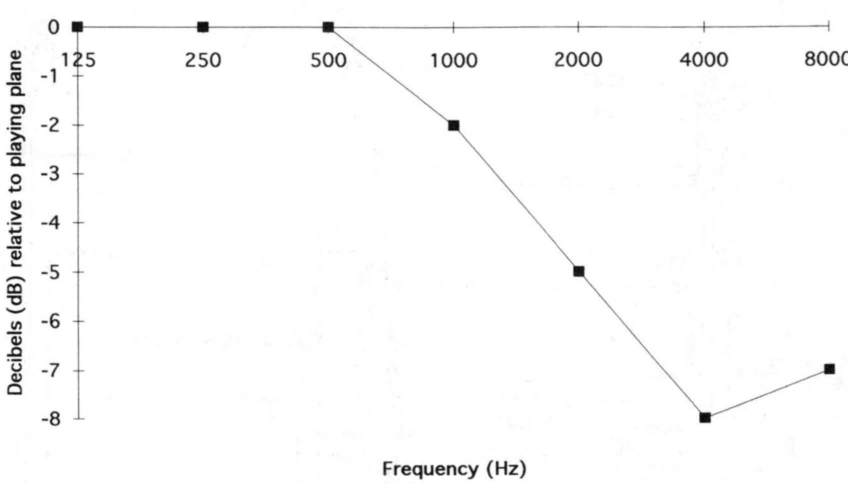

Figure 4–7. The directional characteristics of a trumpet if measured on the playing plane and if measured at 45° below the playing plane. (From "Four Environmental Techniques to Reduce the Effect of Music Exposure on Hearing," by M. Chasin & J. Chong, 1995, *Medical Problems of Performing Artists, 10,* p. 67. Copyright 1995 by Hanley & Belfus, Inc. Adapted with permission.)

from reaching the musicians directly in front of them. More specific information regarding this feature of belled instruments will be discussed in Chapter 8.

Since high frequencies are highly directional (away from the musician), they may not be heard well by the trumpet player such that the phonemic spectrum is probably more low-frequency in nature than the measured phonetic spectrum. Ear protection that serves to attenuate high-frequency sounds, possibly due to the proximity to a percussion section with cymbals and gongs, may be beneficial for trumpet players.

Bowed Stringed Instruments

These instruments comprise the violin, the viola, the cello, and the bass. Figure 4–8 shows the essential physical makeup of a violin—the smallest member of the bowed stringed family.

Helmholtz was instrumental in defining the physical behavior of the bowing mechanism. When the bow (with rosin) is drawn across the string, the string is drawn sideways until the tension of the string overcomes the attraction of the bow and rosin. At this point the string swings back and is again picked up by the bow. An analogous situation is observed when one draws one's fingernails across a blackboard.

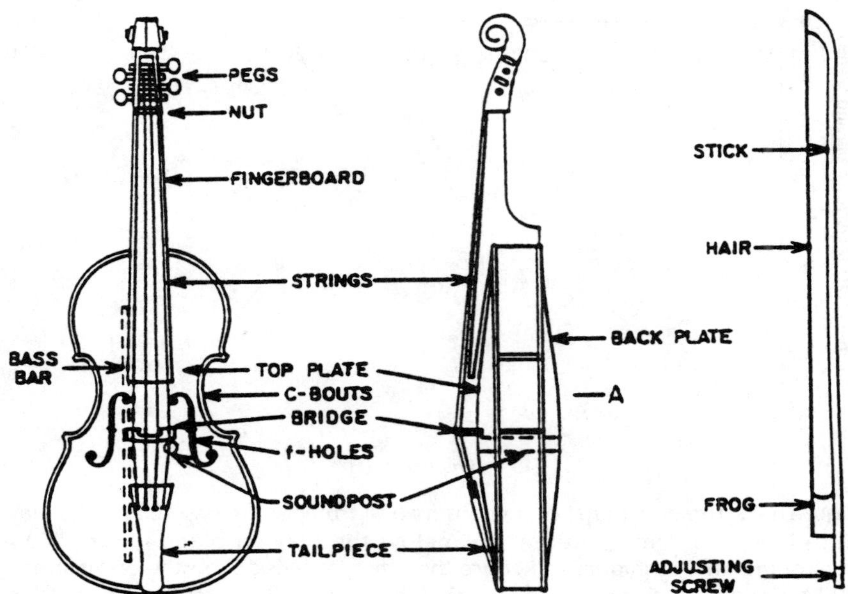

Figure 4–8. The essential parts of the violin and bow. (From *The Acoustical Foundations of Music* [p. 190], by J. Backus, 1977, New York: W. W. Norton & Company, Inc. Copyright 1977 by W. W. Norton & Company, Inc. Reprinted with permission.)

Stringed instruments are articulated with the musician's fingers on the neck in order to shorten the effective length of the string. Such articulation tends to dampen the string's vibration, with a slight reduction in playing intensity. To assess the most intense sound that can be played (see Chapter 6), an open string note is usually the most appropriate. Frequently, a musician may wish to cause a small oscillation of the string's fundamental frequency. This oscillation is called *vibrato* (approximately 6 Hz) and serves to break up standing wave patterns in the performing venue as well as to add richness to the music.

Like the piano, the strings are under a high degree of tension (approximately 25 kg) and are held tightly at both ends of the instrument. Sound vibrations from the strings are transduced to the soundboard by the bridge. Holes shaped in the letter "f" on either side of the strings allow for air vibrations to escape. These "f holes" are also used to alter the formants of the instrument by the manufacturer.

The interior of a violin is not as symmetrical as the exterior. The bridge footplate for the treble strings is connected to a soundpost, which in turn connects the frònt and back plates of the violin. The soundpost serves to aid in the transduction of the sound as well as for physical support. The bass side of the bridge footplate transduces sound to a bass bar that runs the length of the top plate of the violin.

Stringed instruments have three major formants. The air enclosed by the violin possesses an "air resonance," the vibrational characteristics of the wood of the violin has a "wood resonance," and the bridge itself has a broadly tuned high-frequency resonance. There is typically a cutoff point above the bridge-associated resonance that limits the high-frequency transduction of these instruments. It is thought that the difference between a priceless Stradivarius and a more modest violin relates to the nature of the wood resonance. Table 4–3 summarizes these resonances for the violin, the viola, and the cello.

The strings of the these instruments are tuned in fifths (i.e., a difference of 5 white notes on the piano keyboard) and care is taken by manufacturers to ensure that the various resonances coincide with one or more of the fundamental frequencies of the strings. For example, in the violin the four strings are G_3, D_4, A_4, and E_5. The D_4 string corresponds to the second mode of the air resonance and the A_4 string corresponds to the second mode of the wood resonance. This serves to enhance the playing intensity of these instruments.

The viola tends to be more varied in construction than the violin and is tuned a fifth lower, with strings at C_3, G_3, D_4, and A_4. The cello strings are tuned a full octave lower than the viola at C_2, G_2, D_3, and A_3.

Because a violin only has a 30 dB dynamic range (from pianissimo to fortissimo), orchestras employ a large number of violinists. It is impossible for each and every violin to be in perfect pitch with each other and there will be a small range of frequencies played for each note. This spreading of the notes is referred to as the *chorus effect* and accounts for the "richness" that a string section usually possesses.

Although the maximum levels of the cello and bass are not excessive, peak sound levels measured at a violinist's or violist's left ear can exceed 110 dB SPL (and are rarely less than 80 dB SPL).

Table 4–3. Formants for Violin, Viola, and Cello

Instrument	Air Resonance	Wood Resonance	Bridge Resonance
Violin	290 Hz	440 Hz	3000–3500 Hz
Viola	230 Hz	350 Hz	2000 Hz ?
Cello	125 Hz	175 Hz	2000 Hz

Unlike reeded woodwind instruments, string players need to hear the magnitude of the upper harmonics in order to be musically satisfied. There are many cases of wrist or arm damage in violinists who are placed under poorly constructed performance pit overhangs that absorb the higher frequency energy components. Violinsts tend to bow harder to compensate for this loss of high-frequency information in an attempt to re-establish the harmonic content. Figure 4–9 shows the spectrum generated by a violinist who was placed under a poorly constructed overhang and the spectrum of an unobstructed note. These musicians frequently report right arm and wrist strain resulting from "overbowing" their instrument.

Chapter 8 will present a further discussion regarding potential injuries related to a desire for a proper balance between perceptive requirements and the acoustic output of the instrument.

Percussion Instruments

There are a large number of percussion instruments ranging from gongs and bars, to the glockenspiel and the tympani. Large sections of textbooks have been written on the acoustics of percussion instruments, and the interested reader is referred to Campbell and Greated (1987) for an excellent overview.

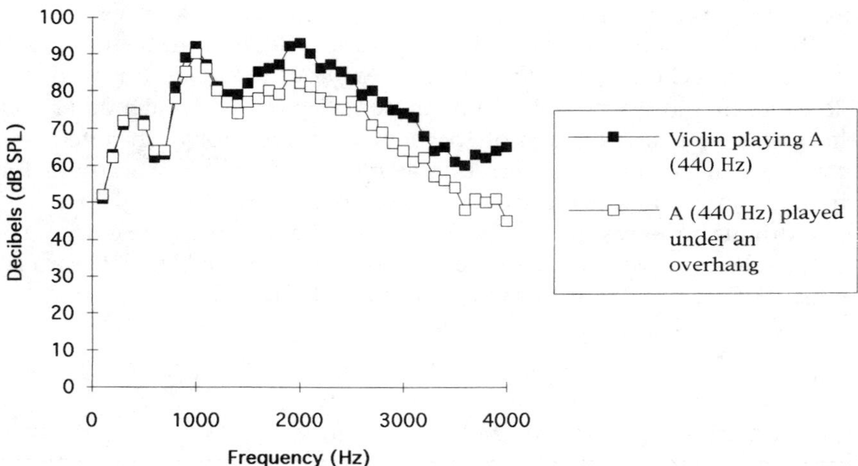

Figure 4–9. Effect on the spectrum of A_4 (440 Hz) of a poorly constructed overhang as compared with no overhang. (From "Four Environmental Techniques to Reduce the Effect of Music Exposure on Hearing," by M. Chasin & J. Chong, 1995, *Medical Problems of Performing Artists, 10,* p. 68. Copyright 1995 by Hanley & Belfus, Inc. Reprinted with permission.)

Rectangular percussive bars and the glockenspiel (a series of tuned bars) are perhaps the instruments that are most easily described. These bars, as used in their normal fashion, behave as one half wavelength resonators, with the ends left free to oscillate. These bars are coupled to a stand at a point approximately one third the distance from either end. There is a node location at these points so minimal damping of the sound occurs. The longer the bar, the lower the frequency that it characterizes. Because bars are one half wavelength resonators, a bar that is double the length of another will have a frequency that is one octave lower.

Cymbals, gongs, and drumheads have complex modes of vibration on their surfaces that characterize the pitch of the instrument. Symphonic hand held cymbals exhibit an interesting characteristic in that the sound level can be greater one second after hitting them together than when initially hit. Depending on their size, cymbals can have energy over 6000 Hz (see Figure 8–5).

The tympani (or kettledrum) is a metal hemisphere (usually made of copper) with a 0.2 mm cover of plastic or calfskin over the top. At the bottom of the hemisphere is a vent hole that functions to equalize the air pressure inside of the tympani to the barometric air pressure in the performance hall. This vent also has an acoustic function by completely damping out the first mode of resonance of the tympani, such that it is tuned to its second mode of resonance. For the 28" and 25" diameter tympanis typically found in many orchestral environments, the frequency ranges from F_2 (87 Hz) to F_3 (174 Hz).

The Human Voice

Most of the development of the source–formant filter–radiation model shown in Figure 4–1a was derived from work on the human voice and vocal tract. Like most of the nonpercussive instruments discussed above, a vibrating (glottal) source of evenly spaced harmonics functions as the input to the vocal tract resonator. The physics of the vocal chord vibration are similar to that of the reed in the clarinet and are related to the interplay between the Bernoulli principle (see Chapter 3) drawing the vocal chords together and the subglottal pressure forcing them apart. The rate of movement of the vocal chords caused by this interplay is called the fundamental frequency and is usually denoted by f_0. This rate defines the pitch of the speaker (or singer). The amplitude of this harmonic complex falls off exponentially ($1/N^2$), with frequency relative to that of the fundamental.

The vocal tract resonator (unlike that of stringed instruments) can be changed by articulators such as the tongue, lips, soft palate, and degree of mouth opening. In its simplest (yet still sufficient) form the vocal tract can be thought of as a tube that is closed at one end (the vocal chords) and open at the other (open mouth for vowels). For vowels, the vocal tract then can be thought of as a quarter wavelength resonator, with odd number multiples of the formants or resonances. The resonant behavior becomes more complex when the tongue creates a constriction in the oral cavity. Helmholtz resonances are established by the constriction (between the body of the tongue and roof of mouth) and the volume of air behind the constriction. The nasal cavity introduces additional wavelength resonances as well as half wavelength antiresonances. It is this highly versatile resonator that allows for human communication. Figure 4–10 shows a stylized human vocal tract.

Like woodwinds and stringed instruments (but unlike brass instruments), the behavior of the glottal source is independent of the vocal tract configuration. One's pitch can change as one sings a scale, but as long as the vocal tract configuration is kept constant, the formant pattern will not change.

When articulating or singing bass notes (with a low-frequency fundamental frequency) the voice is referred to as "mellow" or "rich." A low-pitched voice, such as one with a fundamental frequency of 100 Hz, would have a harmonic structure with energy spaced every 100 Hz (i.e., 100 Hz, 200 Hz, 300 Hz, . . .), and many harmonics would contribute to the formation of the resonant or formant structure. For a vowel such as [a] as in "father" with its first formant at 500 Hz, there would be five harmonics defining the spectral envelope up to 500 Hz. However, for a falsetto voice (f_0 = 400 Hz) only one harmonic element would be available to define the first formant. As a result high-pitched voices such as a falsetto or soprano tend to be less intelligible than a more bass voice.

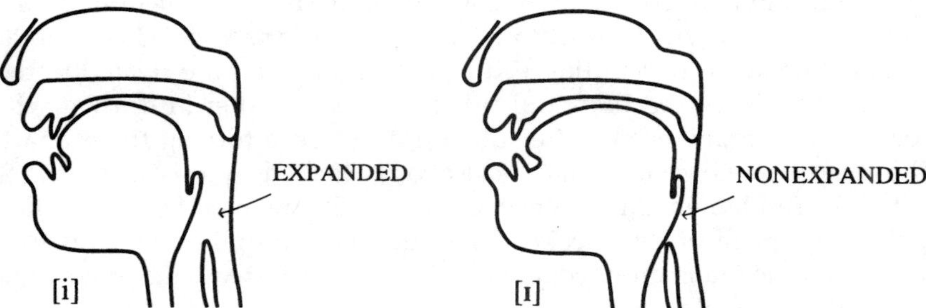

Figure 4–10. Stylized human vocal tract showing both an expanded and a nonexpanded larynx. (From *Theoretical and Practical Phonetics* [p. 188] by H. E. Rogers, 1991, Mississauga, Ontario: Copp Clark Pitman Ltd. Copyright by Copp Clark Pitman Ltd. Reprinted with permission.)

Indeed it was this rationale that led television and radio stations to hire only male announcers in the early days of the respective media. As it turns out, though, a female's fundamental frequency is only slightly higher than that of a male's and females tend to have slightly higher frequency formants due to their shorter vocal tract, so a roughly equal number of harmonics define the formant structure for a woman's voice.

The bass and baritone singers have a low-pitched voice, with a fundamental frequency ranging from approximately E_2 (83 Hz) to F_4 (350 Hz). These limits vary widely depending on singer and skill level.

A question arises with bass and baritone singers who are backed by an orchestra. How can these singers be heard over the background of the orchestra music? The long-term averaged spectrum of an orchestra is not all that different from that of a low-pitched human voice. The bass and baritone singers use three methods to accomplish this. The first is that they use short sharp puffs of air through the larynx, which emphasizes the higher frequency harmonics. The second is the use of vibrato, which is approximately 5–7 Hz (Titze, 1995). The third is the use of the singer's formant.

The *singer's formant* is the generation of an extra formant in the 2500–3000 Hz region and is created by the intentional widening of a 2 cm long portion of the vocal tract just above the larynx (i.e., the larynx tube). This has also been referred to as an *expanded larynx* (shown in Figure 4–10) and forms the basis for a feature that is linguistically distinctive in several West African languages (Lindau, 1978). The singer's formant can be 12–15 dB more intense than the surrounding orchestra and significantly improves the high-frequency signal-to-noise ratio.

Classically trained soprano singers can have a fundamental frequency up to 800 Hz and can generate levels in excess of 115 dB SPL. Nonclasssically trained sopranos can generate only 105–110 dB SPL, with very few exceptions. It is an important question to ask whether a soprano singer is classically trained, as this may indicate a possibility of a self-induced hearing loss.

Sopranos use a technique called *formant tuning* to enhance their intensity and dynamic range. There is no inherent reason why a harmonic should coincide with a formant other than coincidence. However, many sopranos and some tenors can subtly alter the configuration of their vocal tracts to move a formant to the same frequency as one of their harmonics, thus significantly improving audibility when backed by an orchestra. Figure 4–11 shows the relative importance of the singer's formant and formant tuning for the different registers of singers.

SUMMARY

The clinically efficient assessment of the spectral characteristics of a musical instrument is facilitated by an expectation of its spectral shape,

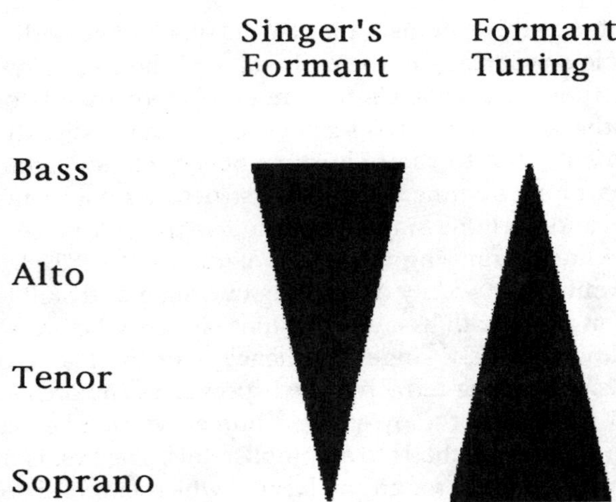

Figure 4–11. Relative importance of the singer's formant and formant tuning for the different registers of singers.

just as a knowledge of acoustics facilitates the analysis of speech in a speech spectrogram.

Seven classes of musical instruments were described, based on the development of physical principles established in Chapter 3. These include the piano, woodwinds, flute, brass, strings, percussion, and the human voice.

A distinction was made between the phonetic and the phonemic spectra. A phonetic spectrum is the measured energy output and the phonemic spectrum is an interpretation based on the perceptive requirements of musicians in their particular instrument category.

The source–formant filter–radiation model was introduced, showing three independent aspects of the production of the sound spectrum. The only exception to this model is the brass instrument, where a feedback loop affects the nature of the sound source.

CHAPTER
5

Hearing Protection

INTRODUCTION

Hearing protection was historically used first in the "high tech" fields such as the aircraft industry and later in a more general industrial "low tech" environment. The industrial usage initially resulted in a "one size fits all" philosophy regardless of input noise spectrum; however, as more became understood about hearing protection and its relationship to hearing in noise, the specifications became more appropriate.

Musicians are the extreme case of a high tech industry. The requirements among musicians vary widely and the tolerance for a less than optimal attenuation response is understandably quite low.

This chapter will cover the following:

1. overview of the attenuation characteristics of hearing protection
2. acoustically tuned hearing protection
3. optimal musician hearing protection
4. electronic based hearing protection
5. assessment techniques
6. single value attenuation rating schemes
7. other "hearing protectors."

OVERVIEW OF ATTENUATION CHARACTERISTICS

Many studies have examined the bases for the maximum attenuation levels from hearing protection (Zwislocki, 1953, 1957; Shaw & Theissen, 1958, 1962; Berger, 1986). These factors pertain not only to the thickness and density of the material used in hearing protectors, but also to the level of bone-conducted sound transmission. Berger, in reviewing the methods to assess the attenuation of hearing protectors, noted that at 2000 Hz, the bone conduction limit for hearing protection was the lowest (40 dB). That is, attenuations of greater than 40 dB in the 2000 Hz region are artifacts of the "objective" measuring system. At this level, sound is conducted through the temporal bone directly to the cochlea, bypassing the air conduction route. One can measure an attenuation in excess of 40 dB at 2000 Hz by the use of artificial test fixtures (ATF) or by a real ear probe microphone measurement technique (such as microphone-in-real-ear [MIRE]), but these values would not correspond with subjective performance. The only exception would be the work of Schroeter (1986), where he constructed an ATF with as much inherent self-insertion loss as possible, and then accounted for the bone conduction route by post-measurement computational corrections. Figure 5–1 is from Berger and shows the bone conduction limits across frequency for hearing protector attenuation.

Closely related to this is the level of the *occlusion effect*. Discussed in more detail in Chapter 6, this effect is the improvement of the lower frequency bone conduction thresholds upon occlusion of the ear canal. This results in the amplification of internal physiological noise that masks the low-frequency unoccluded thresholds (Berger & Kerivan, 1983). The essential characteristics of this phenomenon were first delineated by Zwislocki in the 1950s (Zwislocki, 1953, 1957). Figure 5–2 is from Berger (1988) and shows how the occlusion effect varies with the volume of air enclosed between the hearing protector and the ear drum.

The occlusion effect is well known in the hearing aid field and typically results in an echoey sensation being reported by hearing aid users. Extending the bore of the hearing aid canal into the bony portion of the external ear canal can reduce the occlusion effect. As discussed in Chapter 6, the extent of the occlusion effect can be measured clinically with the use of real ear measurement equipment as well as by hand-held occlusion effect meters.

Another feature of hearing protection is that, unless specifically designed, higher frequency sounds are attenuated more than the lower frequency sounds.

Figure 5–3 shows the frequency-dependent characteristics of a typical industrial foam plug deeply inserted into the ear canal. Two acoustic phenomena account for the frequency dependence and these have both been introduced and discussed in Chapter 3.

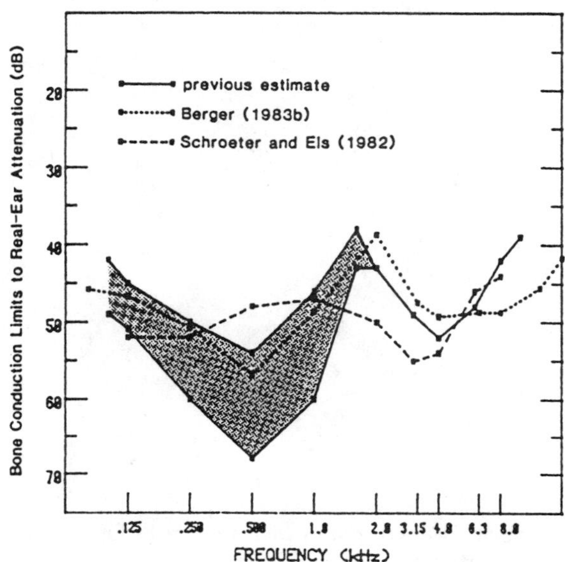

Figure 5–1. The bone conduction limits across frequency for hearing protector attenuation. (From "Methods of Measuring the Attenuation of Hearing Protection Devices," by E. H. Berger, 1986, *Journal of the Acoustical Society of America, 79,* p. 1673. Copyright 1986 by the American Institute of Physics. Reprinted with permission.)

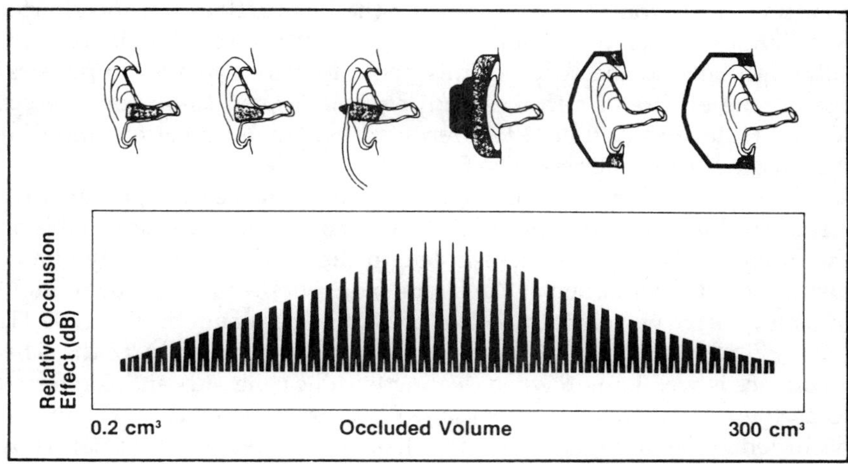

Figure 5–2. The occlusion effect varies with the volume of air enclosed between the ear protector and the ear drum. (From "Tips for Fitting Hearing Protectors," by E. H. Berger, 1988, *E•A•R•LOG 19*. Copyright 1988 by Cabot Safety Corporation. Reprinted with permission.)

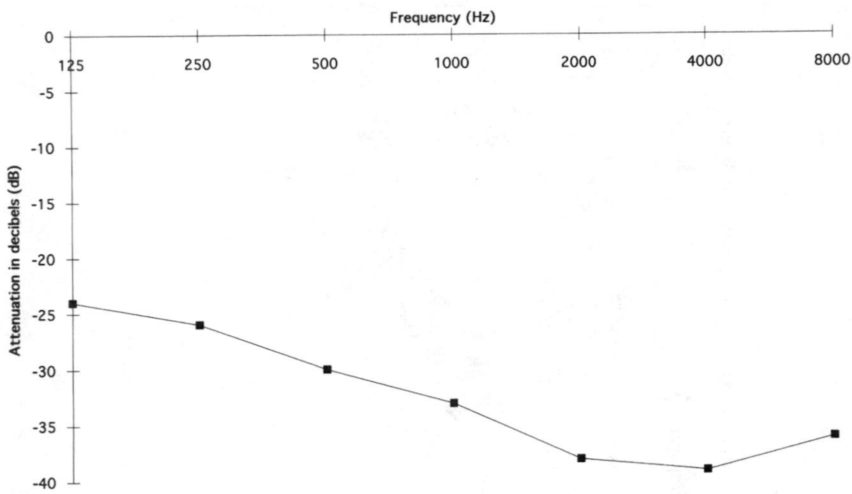

Figure 5–3. Attenuation characteristics of a typical industrial foam earplug that is deeply inserted into the ear canal.

The first phenomenon is that all frequencies whose one half wavelength is less than the diameter of the obstruction (or hearing protector) are attenuated. Low-frequency sounds (i.e., long wavelengths) are acoustically "myopic" and do not see the obstruction, but the shorter wavelength higher frequency sounds acoustically see the obstruction. Although beyond the scope of this book, to fully explain the physical issues, the effects of stiffness and mass also need to be considered. Nixon, Hille, and Kettler (1967) reported essentially no attenuation for the very low-frequency sounds (from 30 to 100 Hz).

The second phenomenon pertains to the existence of a quarter wave resonator due to the presence of the ear canal. The human ear canal is on the order of 25 mm (one inch) in length that is closed at the tympanic membrane side and open at the lateral side. Such a tube can be thought of as a quarter wavelength resonator with a frequency in the 2700 Hz region. The magnitude of the resonance is approximately 17 dB. This resonance is well known when dealing with hearing aids and is referred to as the *real ear unaided response* (REUR). Whenever the ear canal is occluded (with a hearing aid or a hearing protector), this naturally occurring resonance is lost. Plugging the ear canal is acoustically comparable to a musician inserting his or her hand into the bell of the French horn. With earplugs, an additional high-frequency (insertion) loss is caused by this destruction of the 2700 Hz resonance.

In contrast, earmuffs do not destroy the natural ear resonance in the 2700 Hz region, and as such there is less relative high-frequency attenuation than if earplugs were used. Earmuffs do, however, yield greater attenuations in the 500–1000 Hz region. As an additional side effect, as can be observed in Figure 5–2, the level of the occlusion effect will be less with large volume earmuffs than with many earplug fittings.

One cannot, however, state definitively that the use of earmuffs yield improved intelligibility in noise over that of the use of earplugs, since hearing loss configuration and large subject variability are confounding factors (Abel, Alberti, Haythornwaite, & Riko, 1982).

ACOUSTICALLY TUNED EAR PROTECTION ALTERNATIVES

Both a significant occlusion effect and the frequency-dependent characteristic of hearing protection can be disasterous for musicians. The occlusion effect can be utilized in some cases (see Chapters 6 and 8) to benefit the musician, but as a general rule, this phenomenon should be minimized. There is rarely a case of the frequency-dependent characteristic of hearing protection being beneficial for any musician (except with certain types of percussion instruments).

Killion, Stewart, Falco, and Berger (1988) devised a custom earplug with approximately 15 decibels of attenuation over a wide range of frequencies. This was based on earlier work of Elmer Carlson. The earplug, named the ER-15™ (manufactured by Etymotic Research, Inc.), has become widely accepted by musicians as well as some industrial workers who work in relatively quiet environments. Figure 5–4 shows the attenuation characteristics of the ER-15 earplug along with the ER-25™ earplug, the vented/tuned earplug, and an industrial-type foam plug (from Figure 5–3) for comparison purposes. Figure 5–4 is also found in Appendix I. Figure 5–5 shows the effect the ER-15 has on the spectrum of a violin [A_4 (440 Hz)] played at a mezzo forte level. Note that the attenuated spectrum is essentially parallel to the unattenuated one.

The design of the ER-15 earplug (and its partner, the ER-25 earplug that provides approximately 25 decibels of uniform attenuation) is remarkably simple. Essentially, a button-sized element that functions as an acoustic compliance is connected to a custom ear mold, with the volume of air in the sound bore acting as an acoustic mass. The resulting resonance between the compliance and the mass is in the 2700 Hz region and is designed to offset the insertion loss caused by the earplug. The high-frequency resonance is sufficiently broad to compensate for the relative high-frequency attenuation. Because the ER-element is manufactured in the factory, the compliance value is constant. Ear mold labora-

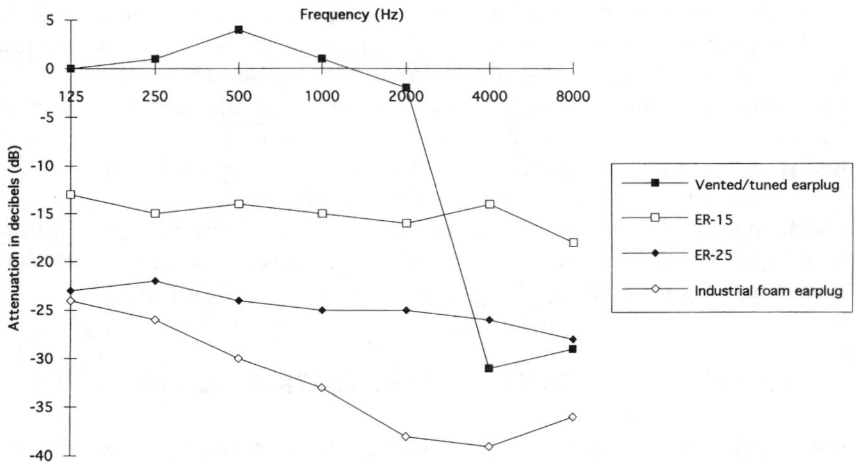

Figure 5–4. Attenuation characteristics of the ER-15, ER-25, and the vented/tuned earplugs. The industrial earplug data is also given for comparison purposes. (From "A Clinically Efficient Hearing Protection Program for Musicians," by M. Chasin & J. Chong, 1992, *Medical Problems of Performing Artists, 7,* p. 41. Copyright 1992 by Hanley & Belfus, Inc. Adapted with permission.)

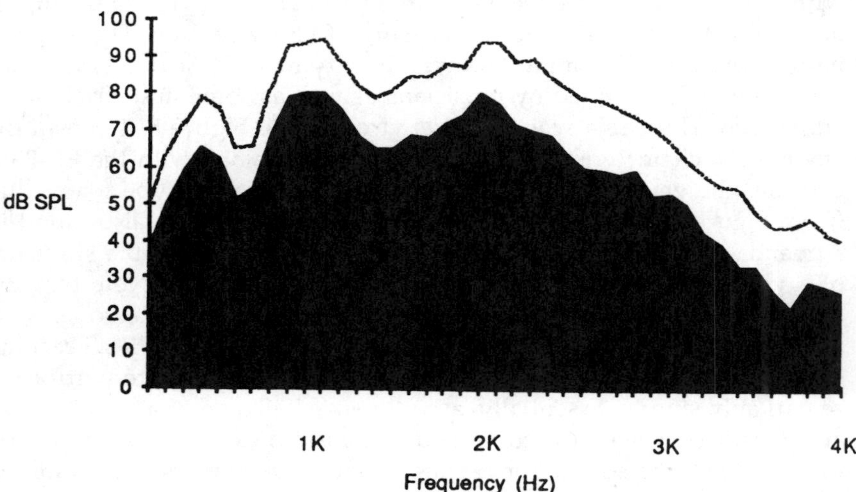

Figure 5–5. The effect of the ER-15 earplug on the spectrum of a violin playing the note A_4 (440 Hz). The attenuated spectrum is parallel to the unattenuated one bottom/black. (From "A Clinically Efficient Hearing Protection Program for Musicians," by M. Chasin & J. Chong, 1992, *Medical Problems of Performing Artists, 7,* p. 42. Copyright 1992 by Hanley & Belfus, Inc. Reprinted with permission.)

tories use a "mass meter" to verify that the custom ear mold has the correct volume of air in the sound bore in order to establish an essentially flat attenuation pattern. A schematic and ER-15 is shown in Figure 5–6.

Because the ear mold is a custom-made product, the length of the sound bore can be made as long as possible. As pointed out by Zwislocki (1957) as well as is shown in Figure 5–2, the deeper the end of the ear mold in the ear canal, the less the occlusion effect. Research with completely-in-the-canal (CIC) hearing aids indicates that this can be clinically achieved if the mold terminates 2–3 mm inside of the bony portion of the ear canal (Chasin, 1994).

A noncustom (and less expensive) product is also available called the ER-20/HI-FI earplug (Killion, Stewart, Falco, & Berger, 1992) and essentially uses the folded horn concept to enhance the higher frequencies and thereby reduce the high-frequency attenuation. The folded horn concept is a modification of the acoustic transformer effect discussed in Chapter 3, where the flaring tube is folded on itself because of space limitations but the high-frequency enhancement is maintained. This idea was used unsuccessfully in the mid 1980s to obtain some of the horn benefits for in-the-ear hearing aids (Gauthier & Burak, 1983). The other purpose of the folded horn is to relocate the sound entry point for the earplug from a position about 15 mm outside the entrance of the ear canal to the floor of the concha where there is significant high-frequency amplification.

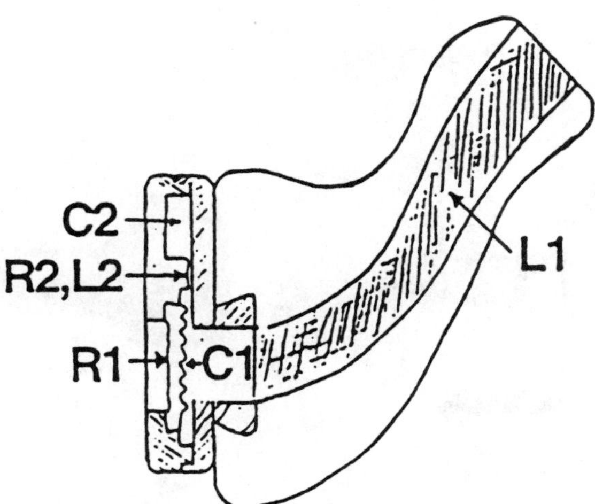

Figure 5–6. A schematic of the ER-15 custom-molded flat attenuation earplug. See text for explanation. C = compliance; R = resistance; L = inductance. (Courtesy of Etymotic Research.)

Figure 5–7 shows the ER-20/HI-FI earplug. This earplug has a noise reduction rating (NRR) of 12 dB, and a new version with an NRR of 16 dB is also available. Unlike the ER-15 and ER-25 earplugs, the ER-20/HI-FI earplug has a slight high-frequency roll-off with attenuations ranging from 15 dB for the lower frequency sounds to 22 dB for the higher frequency sounds.

The ER-series of earplugs can be modified for those musicians with unusual ear canal resonances (not 2700 Hz) or for those with unusual hearing requirements, possibly due to a mild hearing loss.

In order to provide the theoretical basis for the clinical modification of the ER-series of earplugs, one can also view the mass of air in the earplug sound bore as an inductance (*L*). The resonant frequency of this system can be given as being proportional to the square root of the inductance (*L*) over the compliance (C). The compliance (C) is a constant and is set by the design of the attenuator button. However, the inductance (*L*) is proportional to the length of the sound bore and inversely proportional to the cross-sectional area of the sound bore. The summarizing equation is shown in Figure 5–8.

With this equation as a tool, it becomes clear how the earplug changes can affect the frequency response. To increase the resonant frequency, one needs to increase the inductance (*L*). This can be accomplished by increasing the length and/or decreasing the diameter of the

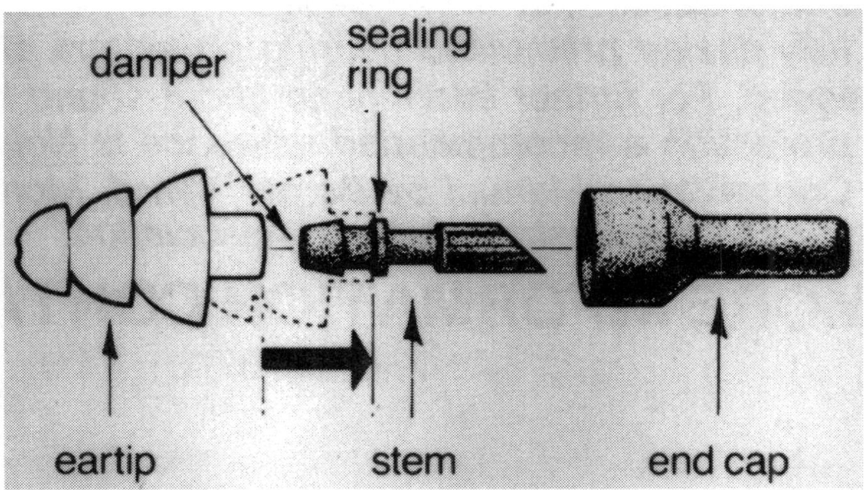

Figure 5–7. The design of the ER-20/HI-FI noncustom earplug. (Courtesy of Etymotic Research.)

$$F_{res} \ \alpha \ \sqrt{(L/C)}$$

$$\text{where } L \ \alpha \ (\text{Length/cross-sectional area})$$

Figure 5–8. Equation relating the resonant frequency (*F*) to the inductance (*L*) and the compliance (*C*).

bore. Not only would the resonant frequency of the system be higher, there would also be less high-frequency attenuation. Such a modification would be useful for musicians with a slight high-frequency music-induced hearing loss who do not require significant high-frequency attenuation.

To decrease the resonant frequency, one needs to decrease the inductance (*L*) by decreasing the bore length and/or increasing the diameter of the bore. Associated with a lower resonant frequency would also be more high-frequency attenuation than in the nonmodified ER-series earplug. Figure 5–9 shows the effect of modifying the ER-15 earplug, expressed as an attenuation from the unplugged condition (REUR). The nonmodified attenuation characteristics of the ER-15 earplug are also shown for comparison. It should be emphasized that the ER-series of earplugs will cease to become flat or uniform atttenuators when the dimensions of the earplug are altered beyond that specified by the ear mold laboratory's mass meter readings.

Another approach to acoustic tuning of hearing protection takes a different slant. Instead of attempting to uniformly attenuate the music, an earplug can be constructed that has minimal acoustic effect in the lower frequencies and a significant high-frequency attenuation. This category has been termed the vented/tuned earplug (Chasin & Chong, 1991, 1992, 1994) and is ideal for many bass and some woodwind musical instruments. The vent/tuned earplug is custom made with a select-a-vent (SAV) drilled down the main sound bore. In its most open position, it is acoustically transparent below 2000 Hz (one octave below the top note on the piano keyboard), with a significant high-frequency attenuation (up to maximum of 28 dB—with a typical attenuation of 20 dB). It can easily be simulated by removing the attenuator button on the ER-series of earplugs.

Many musicians are in an environment that has very little low frequency energy that could be considered damaging, but have to sit near a high-frequency source. An example may be a clarinet player who sits in front of the percussion cymbal or a trumpet section.

A vented/tuned earplug would allow the clarinet player to hear his or her own music but provide significant attenuation for the high frequency stimuli in the immediate vicinity.

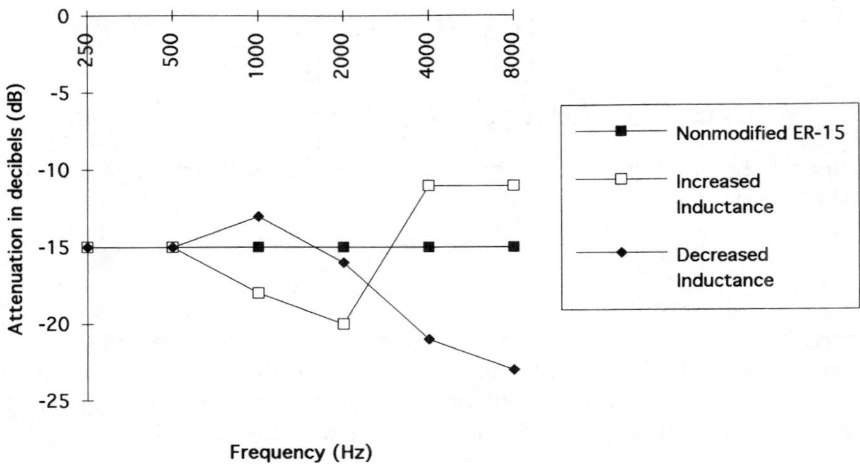

Figure 5–9. Attenuation characteristics of modifying the ER-15 by altering the inductance (*L*).

Placing the SAV covers over the sound bore would increase the overall attenuation, ultimately creating the equivalent of an industrial earplug. The vast majority of musicians use this earplug in the completely open position, and the attenuation pattern of the vented/tuned earplug is shown in Figure 5–4. There is a small (4–5 dB) resonance in the 500 Hz region. This is an acoustic inertance and is caused by the mass of air in the "vent" vibrating. Such a resonance is frequently observed in the study of hearing aids and has been termed a *vent-associated resonance.* As will be seen in Chapters 6 and 8, this small resonance can be used to improve the monitoring ability of some musicians and some vocalists. It also can be used as part of a program to reduce vocal nodules; this will be further discussed in Chapter 8.

Modifications of the vented/tuned earplugs are also available that use acoustic resistors in, or in front of, the vent. Ear mold laboratories have different names for these "filtered" vented/tuned earplugs, and the attenuation characteristics will vary depending on the filter used as well as on the sound bore dimensions.

OPTIMAL MUSICIAN HEARING PROTECTION

Chapter 4 discussed the spectral characteristics of various musical instruments as well as their perceptive requirements. Understandably the optimal hearing protection for one musician may be different for another. Given the hearing protection alternatives provided in the last section, what are the best hearing protectors for each musician group? Table 5–1 shows a list of musician groups, the most probable source of noise exposure, and the hearing protector of choice.

Most of the rationale was provided in Chapter 3, but some explanation is necessary. It is occasionally not clear that one hearing protector is better than another, and it may be clinically wise to try one and then another to obtain the optimal result. This can be accomplished by a specification of the ER-15 earplugs, and a trial with the attenuator button and then without (i.e., vented/tuned earplugs). In those few cases where the proper hearing protection is not clear, without going to great expense, the ER-20/HI-FI earplug may be used and contrasted with a foam industrial earplug with a 3 mm vent drilled down the center, held open by a short length of standard #13 hearing aid tubing. However, in

Table 5–1. Optimal Hearing Protection for Musicians

Instrument	Auditory Damage	Earplugs
Reeded woodwinds	Brass section to rear	ER-15 Vented/tuned
Flutes	Flutes (>105 dB SPL)	ER-15 Vented/tuned
Small strings	Small strings (>110 dB SPL)	ER-15
Large strings	Brass section to rear	Vented/tuned
Brass	Brass	Vented/tuned
Percussion	Percussion (high hats)	ER-25
Vocalists Solo	Soprano (>115 dB SPL)	Vented/tuned
Nonsolo	Other instruments	ER-15
Amplified Instruments	Speakers/monitors	ER-15

most cases, Table 5–1 prescribes a fairly accurate hearing protector. A copy of Table 5–1 is also given in Appendix I.

Many of the reeded woodwinds (clarinets, oboes, bassoons, and saxophones) are situated in front of the trumpet section or the percussion section. The reeded woodwind musicians need to hear the lower frequency interresonant notes of their instruments in order to play properly. Generally, good audibility of the high-frequency sounds is not required. Use of a vented/tuned earplug would be ideal in these cases. However, on some occasions, these musicians may play in a jazz or blues band and require a broader band earplug because of the amplified nature of the music. Use of the ER-15 earplug may become necessary.

Flutes players can generate peak levels in excess of 105 dB SPL (and in excess of 120 dB SPL for piccolo players). The ER-15 earplug is the primary choice. In cases where there is an audiometric asymmetry (typically with the right ear being worse), a vented/tuned earplug will be optimal with a 2 mm vent on the better ear and a 3 mm vent on the worse ear. This innovation will serve to balance the high-frequency hearing, which appears to be quite important for most flute players (more so than any other musician category).

The small string players are the violinists and the violists. It is crucial for these musicians to maintain the relative balance between the low-frequency fundamental energy and the higher frequency harmonics. Because peak levels can be in excess of 110 dB SPL, the ER-15 is the hearing protector of choice.

The large string players comprise the bass, cello, and harp. It is extremely rare that these instruments can generate levels in excess of 85 dB SPL; however, the auditory damage may derive from the brass section to their rear. The hearing protector of choice is the vented/tuned earplug, in its most open position. The full harmonic spectrum of these instruments will be audible while significantly attenuating the high-frequency energy components from the trumpet section behind them.

The brass players, interestingly enough, are not very prone to hearing loss from their instruments. Brass players are usually situated in the rear, and as discussed in Chapter 4, most of the damaging energy of their instruments is directed away from them. Use of the vented/tuned earplugs may be advisable if the players are situated "downwind" from other brass instruments or behind the French horn section. In some cases where these musicians play in rock or jazz bands, the ER-15 earplug would be required due to the amplified nature of the music.

Percussion players require more attenuation than that provided by the ER-15 earplug. The ER-25 earplugs were designed with them in mind and provide the correct balance between too little attenuation (with the possibility of an increase in their hearing loss) and too much attenuation (with a loss of monitoring ability).

Solo vocalists may not require any hearing protection. If they are classically trained sopranos, they may be able to generate levels in excess of 115 dB SPL and in some cases be an auditory threat to themselves. This is not a common problem, but eight cases have been documented since 1988. The vented/tuned approach works best due to the small 500 Hz resonance improving the singer's monitoring ability. Vocalists with these earplugs sing at a slightly less intense level that can serve to protect their vocal chords from trauma. Nonsolo vocalists are typically accompanied by amplified instruments that can generate broad-band spectra. The ER-15 is therefore quite useful. Intentionally shortening the length of the bore serves to increase the occlusion effect, thus providing an increased monitoring ability.

Amplified instruments can be very intense, with many peak levels measured in excess of 120 dB SPL. The ER-15 earplug is the hearing protection of choice, with occasional musicians requiring the ER-25 in some environments.

ELECTRONIC BASED HEARING PROTECTION

Several innovations have allowed some forms of hearing protection to be based on electronic characteristics rather than acoustic ones. The first innovation was *active noise reduction* (ANR) and is based on the principle that two identical signals, when added together out of phase, will cancel. While it is difficult to assess a quickly varying signal and generate another with the identical spectrum but 180° out of phase, it is relatively easy task for steady state signals, especially if they are low frequency (i.e., long wavelength). ANR hearing protection has not gained wide acceptance because of its high cost, its limitation to low-frequency attenuation, and up until recently, its limitation to relatively steady state signals.

In contrast, *active sound transmission* hearing protection has had its major use in hunting where optimal hearing of the movement of the prey has to be coupled with optimal hearing protection. A modified hearing aid circuit is typically utilized that allows for amplification at low input levels but attenuation or clipping at higher levels (such as the blast from a gun). An external monitoring microphone is used to assess the environmental noise/music level, and the amplification stages are reduced or disabled completely above a certain preselected level. Electronically based hearing protection of this type has been used for percussion musicians but typically only during practice sessions.

There are some reports in the literature regarding the use of level-dependent circuits such as the K-AMP™ (Killion, 1993), as well as the use of hearing aids that have been turned off (Berger, 1987; Hétu, Tran

Quoc, & Tougas, 1992), and these have been shown to be quite useful for musicians with mild hearing losses, as long as there is no vent (see Figure 6–6). Since most hearing aid fittings utilize an acoustic vent, hearing aids that are to be used in this fashion should be constructed with a select-a-vent. During music exposure, the musician can plug the vent, and open it to the desired degree for everyday speech communication.

ASSESSMENT TECHNIQUES

There are several objective assessment techniques to determine the attenuation of hearing protectors. Berger (1986) pointed out that the term *attenuation* is rather poorly defined and that instead there should be a discussion of insertion loss and noise reduction.

Insertion loss is a similar measure to insertion gain in the hearing aid field in that two consecutive measures are made with miniature microphones. Insertion loss can be assessed objectively using a microphone-in-real-ear (MIRE) technique. Such a technique is analogous to the real-ear-insertion-response (REIR) for hearing aid assessment. One measure is made in the ear canal without the hearing protection and the other is made in the identical location with the hearing protection in place. The difference is the insertion loss. Because the location of the microphone is identical in both conditions, all factors that affect the SPL, other than the decrease in SPL caused by the hearing protector, are subtracted. This measure is further discussed in Chapter 6 and tends to be the most expedicious for clinical use. A potential problem with the insertion loss measure is the inadvertent contribution of the bone conduction route as shown in Figure 5–1. However, when working with musicians and the relatively mild attenuators used, the bone conduction route never becomes a factor.

Noise reduction is a simultaneous measure made by two separate microphones: one being outside of the hearing protector and the other being on the medial side in the ear canal. A noise reduction measure can be affected by the precise location of the microphone in the ear canal as well as by diffraction effects from the external portion of the ear canal. Yet this measure can be useful in high noise environments and can utilize an actual industrial spectrum as the stimulus.

Subjective techniques can be categorized as *threshold-based*, or *supra threshold*. Threshold-based techniques are the oldest and in most cases provide a high degree of reliability. Associated with any subjective technique, the individual's ability to respond is a factor and this contributes an inevitable source of error. For this reason, the standard deviations tend to be higher than for those techniques that utilize an objective microphone-based procedure.

Real ear attenuation at threshold (REAT) is a subjective technique that seeks to assess the change in the hearing threshold of a subject with and without hearing protection. REAT can be assessed under earphones or (binaurally) in the sound field. Two drawbacks of this measure (especially if measured in the sound field) are an inability to attain a quiet enough environment to achieve a true unprotected condition, and low-frequency masking may occur as a result of physiological noise that overstates the degree of low-frequency attenuation. When REAT is assessed under earphones, the first factor is rarely an issue, but corrections need to be made for a slightly smaller volume, as part or all of the concha is occupied by the hearing protector.

Suprathreshold-based techniques tend to have a poorer test–retest reliability than REAT and are not commonly used. These may include measures of midline lateralization, speech reception thresholds, and other psychophysical tests. For an excellent review of these techniques the interested reader is referred to Alberti (1982) and to Berger (1986).

SINGLE VALUE ATTENUATION RATING SCHEMES

Several single number rating schemes are in use throughout the world. The most commonly used scheme in the United States is the Noise Reduction Rating (NRR). Most parts of Europe use an octave band method as well as the ISO recommended Single Number Rating (SNR). (E.H. Berger, personal communication, 1995). Most provinces in Canada use the ABC scheme where hearing protectors are categorized according to a standard (Z94.2-94) into Class A, B, or C depending on their octave band attenuation values and the measured L_{eq}—a time weighted average (Behar & Desormeaux, 1994).

The NRR has been in widespread use since 1979 as a relatively simple method to characterize the attenuation of hearing protectors. The NRR innovation came from the work of Botsford (1973), who found that the environmental noise measured in dBC (dB C-weighted) and the noise level measured in dBA (dB A-weighted), when assessed in the ear canal with the hearing protector in place, was a constant and could be used to characterize the hearing protector.

However, as pointed out by Preves and Pehringer (1983), the NRR calculation made some simplifying assumptions and required the use of various correction factors. The validity of these assumptions has led to some criticism of the NRR technique. One such assumption is that the environmental noise spectrum is a constant pink noise—equal octave band levels across the spectrum.

To understand the potential problem with this assumption, it may be useful to review and compare the C-weighting and A-weighting networks. The C-weighting network is essentially no weighting at all—less than a one-decibel effect up to 6000 Hz. However, the A-weighting network attempts to simulate human hearing sensitivity—a significant low-frequency roll-off of up to 16 decibels at 125 Hz, with no effect at and above 1000 Hz. Thus, if an environmental noise spectrum has significant low-fequency energy, the dBC measure will be much greater than the dBA measure. In contrast, if there is minimal low-frequency noise, there will be minimal difference between a dBA and a dBC noise measurement.

When a comparison is made between a C-weighted measurement and an A-weighted one, a preliminary form of spectral analysis is being performed. Clearly, accepting the NRR without reference to the spectral shape of the environmental noise can be a major source of error.

The work of NIOSH (see Chapter 2) yielded a correction factor of 3 dB in the calculation of the NRR because some workers do not wear their hearing protection properly, as well as for reasons pertaining to the spectral uncertainties just mentioned. Johnson and Nixon (1974) felt that this correction factor should be 5 or 6 dB. As this figure would be subtracted from the calculation, the NRR would be a worst case scenario. The NRR for each hearing protector is a measure based on the results of a number of subjects. Subsequently a two standard deviation pad is also included as "a statistical adjustment so that the mean values are modified to reflect what some larger proportion of the population will actually achieve" (E.H. Berger, personal communication, 1995). This two standard deviation range covers approximately 95% of the population. The NRR formula is given in Figure 5–10.

As can be seen, if the true noise spectrum has no low-frequency energy (as it may be with treble musical instruments), then the first two terms are identical, and the NRR is simply the attenuation and associated wearing and statistical factors. For the musician's ER-15 uniform attenuator earplug, the octave band attenuation is approximately 15 decibels, with the calculated NRR being only 7 dB. Johnson and Nixon (1974) noted that the NRR tends to be artificially high if there is minimal low-frequency attenuation and would be artificially low if there was a flat attenuation characteristic.

Although simplifying measures such as the NRR have made hearing protector characterization easier for the laboratories, the NRR tends to

NRR = N (C-weighted) – N (A-weighted) + attenuation
(A-weighted) – 3 dB – 2 standard deviations

Figure 5–10. The formula for calculating the noise reduction rating (NRR).

be affected by many artifacts when used for a different purpose than originally intended. It is, unfortunately, a widely held view that the higher the NRR, the better the hearing protector. Depending on the noise or music level, the spectral shape, and the individual's communication or musical requirements, this is certainly not the case. Killion (1993) summarized this with a current day fallacy: "Parvum bonum, plus melius," which means "A little is good: More is better."

OTHER "HEARING PROTECTORS"

Other than the use of individual hearing protection, there are frequent uses of nonpersonal hearing protection.

Clear plastic shields are commonly used in many orchestras and some rock groups. Opaque shields are generally not acceptable in orchestras because they can block the view of the musician and the conductor. Opaque shields have been used in some rock groups and are typically used "edge on" such that their presence is not obvious to the audience. Table 5–2 is from Camp and Horstman (1992) and shows the attenuation characteristics of octave band pure tones.

These data are highly dependent on the exact location of measurement behind the shield. Specifically, the data from Table 5–2 were obtained at a distance of seven inches from the shield. Because of reflections, the further one is from the shield, the less will be the attenuation. Camp and Horstman (1992) argue that these data suggest that "free-standing clear plastic shields provide little protection for the musicians

Table 5–2. Octave Band Attenuation of Opaque Shields[a]

Frequency	Without Shields (dB)	With Shields (dB)	Attenuation
63 Hz	72	72	0
125 Hz	73	72	−1
250 Hz	69	71	+2
500 Hz	81	73	−8
1000 Hz	82	73	−9
2000 Hz	86–89	72–77	−13 avg
4000 Hz	86–87	71–74	−15 avg
6000 Hz	80	62–64	−17 avg

[a]Measured at a distance of 7" behind the shields.

(From "Musician Sound Exposure During Performance of Wagner's Ring Cycle," by J. E. Camp & S. W. Horstman, 1992, *Medical Problems of Performing Artists, 7*, p. 37. Copyright 1992 by Hanley & Belfus, Inc. Reprinted with permission.)

downstream from a given sound-generating source, particularly if the shield is not close to the listener and at ear level" (p. 39). However, if the instrument to the rear of the shield has significant high-frequency energy, use of shields may be an excellent idea, especially if used in conjunction with personal hearing protection.

A potential problem with shields is that the musicians "upstream" may have an enhanced music spectra directed toward their ears. For example, a trumpet player to the rear of a shield may receive reflected energy from his or her own trumpet, thus increasing the spectral level. To minimize this, shields should be angled slightly so that no parallel surfaces can inadvertently enhance the sound levels.

Related to artificial clear plastic shields, the human body possesses natural baffles. Depending on the instrument, the human body and head can serve as a baffle. Violin players who hold the violin off to the left hand side receive some right hearing protection from their head. Specifically, all frequencies whose one-half wavelength is less than the diameter of the head are attenuated. This corresponds to approximately 1500 Hz, such that higher frequency sounds are decreased in intensity at the right ear. This natural head baffle effect acounts for the audiometric asymmetry observed with violin players. The same phenomenon accounts for the audiometrically better left ear of the flute player and the better right ear of many right handed rock drummers.

Finally, the Beatles knew what they were doing in the early 1960s when they spawned the "long hair movement." Figure 5–11 shows the attenuation effect of thick hair worn over the ears. Maximum attenuations of 3–5 dB in the mid-frequencies can be achieved. Although 3–5 dB may not be thought of as a large amount of attenuation, this coupled with personal hearing protection can be significant.

SUMMARY

Hearing protectors, unless specifically designed, attenuate the higher frequency sound energy more than lower frequency energy. Because such a nonuniform attenuation characteristic can be less than optimal for the requirements of a musician, acoustically tuned hearing protectors were developed.

These include the ER-15 and the ER-25 earplugs that, as the names suggest, provide a uniform attenuation of 15 dB and 25 dB, respectively. Modifications of these earplugs are clinically possible in order to obtain different attenuation characteristics, but they will lose their uniform attenuation property. Such earplugs are useful for musicians who either play instruments that have a broad band energy spectrum, or those who

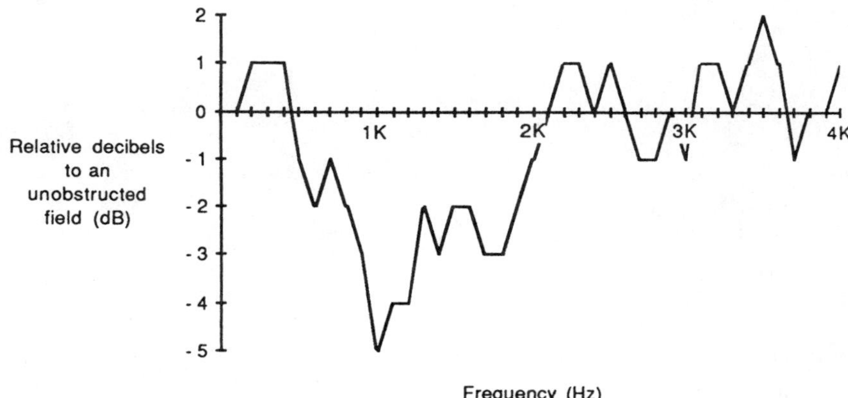

Figure 5–11. Attenuation characteristics of thick hair worn over the ears. (From "A Clinically Efficient Hearing Protection Program for Musicians," by M. Chasin & J. Chong, 1992, *Medical Problems of Performing Artists, 7,* p. 41. Copyright 1992 by Hanley & Belfus, Inc. Reprinted with permission.)

perform in an environment with significant broad band sound energy. The ER-20 (or HI-FI earplug) noncustom earplug is also available.

An alternative, for musicians who require only high-frequency attenuation, is the vented/tuned earplug. An example is a clarinet player who sits in front of a trumpet or percussion section. The specification of the optimal hearing protector is based not only on the musical instrument but on the performing environment musicians may find themselves in.

Custom or noncustom earphones are a useful alternative that allow a musician to listen to live music through individual monitors placed in the person's ear.

Objective techniques such as microphone-in-real-ear (MIRE) and the use of acoustical test fixtures (ATF), and subjective techniques such as REAT are two valid methods for assessing the effects of hearing protection. Regardless of the technique, the resulting data can be expressed in a single number rating scheme such as the Noise Reduction Rating, or NRR.

Other hearing protectors may involve the use of acoustic shields, the acoustic shadow of the musician's own head, and even the slight effect of thick hair worn over the ears.

CHAPTER

6

Clinical Assessment of Musicians— Audiologist as a Detective

INTRODUCTION

A musician's assessment takes a different slant than that of a typical hearing assessment in that it is preventive and educational in nature, rather than diagnostic. It is composed of five distinct parts: (a) case history, (b) audiometric assessment, (c) spectral assessment of the musician's instrument, (d) specification of remedial action, and (e) verification. In a standard hearing assessment, audiometry tends to have the greatest weight. In a musician's assessment, audiometry is typically relegated to a secondary concern.

This chapter can be used as a "cookbook" or a "how to" section. However, as new technology becomes available and different issues gain importance, this chapter will take on the role of merely being a guideline of a general clinical approach. A sample report for a musician is found in Appendix I.

CASE HISTORY

Not all musical instruments generate a sound pressure level that is damaging, even for the most stringent of damage risk criteria (Kryter et al.,

1966). These instruments typically include the reeded woodwinds (clarinet, oboe, and bassoon), the large strings (bass, cello, and harp), piano, nonclassically trained soprano vocalists, and various folk and cultural forms of music.

Nevertheless, many of these musicians do report annoyance from high music levels and in many cases possess music-related high-frequency noise notches in their audiograms. In addition, many musicians with normal audiograms exhibit results on otoacoustic emission tests that suggest noise-induced damage to the outer hair cells in the cochlea (Hall & Santucci, 1995). Damage is known to occur to these outer hair cells before an audiometric loss is observed and can be thought of as an early warning sign of hearing loss (Lonsbury-Martin & Martin, 1990b; Lonsbury-Martin, McCoy, Whitehead, & Martin, 1993).

What then are the causes of such a music-related loss? The audiologist must take a forensic approach. A musician's case history starts with as good a determination as possible of the other sound sources in the musician's environment. The would include both occupational and nonoccupational exposures. Figure 6–1 shows a typical musician's worksheet with the musician denoted as the "X." This is for a vocalist in a rock band. Questions such as "who or what is to your right side?/left side?/rear?/front? . . ." can then be asked with the other sources written or drawn in on the worksheet. Amplifier/speakers, monitors, drums (with a high hat typically on the left side), a brass section, or any other music or sound sources are typical culprits. Note the presence of the drum kit high hat to the left-rear.

If it turns out that there is an audiometric asymmetry consistent with music/noise exposure and which is not expected from the musicians' own instrument, the other sources in the vicinity of the musician become suspect. Further, nonoccupational noise sources such as motorcycles, chain saws, and so on, must also be ruled out as well as other previous band set-up configurations. In the vocalist example in Figure 6–1, a slight audiometric asymmetry in the left ear in the 4000–6000 Hz region could be attributed to the close proximity to the drummer. If the vocalist had spent many years in this environment but is not currently working in that venue, that will be reflected in the counseling and perhaps no recommendations for changes will be made.

Rosenberg (1978) overviewed two case history approaches: the easy conversational approach and the authoritarian approach. The former is rather friendly and is designed to establish rapport, whereas the latter is not unlike a physician's who wants to obtain all the medical information as efficiently as possible. In a typical audiological assessment, the authoritarian approach does seem to glean the required information in a very short time relative to the easy conversational approach and is, therefore, used by most audiologists—hopefully softened with a smile and/or the occasional humorous line.

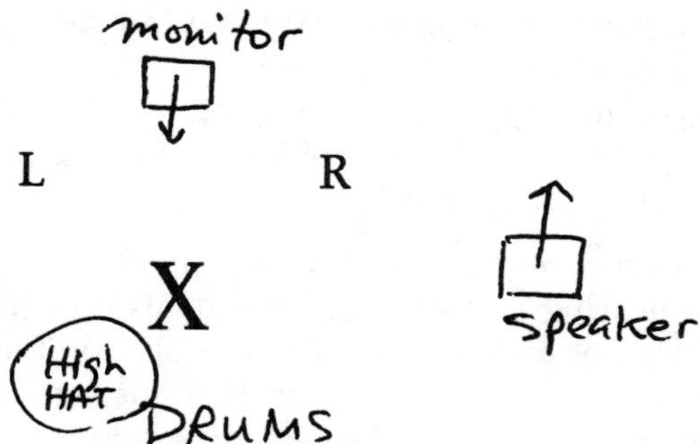

Figure 6–1. Musician's worksheet with the musician (vocalist) denoted by the X. The high hat cymbals are to the left-rear and are a major source of potential music exposure.

The authoritarian approach does, however, assume that we know the sum total of all relevant items that may affect the provisional diagnosis. While to a great extent this is probably the case in the medical model, it is not typically the case with a musician's assessment. Where we may be able to learn and memorize most of the relevant information and relationships among various pieces of medical data, audiologists typically know very little about the life and work of musicians. Therefore an easy conversational approach may be more useful to obtain as much knowledge of the potential noise and/or music sources to which the musician is subject. Using a framework as in Figure 6–1 helps to keep the easy conversational investigative approach on the right track.

Having said this, in addition to standard hearing health medical questions, certain questions should be asked of any person exposed to loud noise. The questions on smoking and general physical health pertain to the information given in Chapter 2 and may increase one's susceptibility to noise exposure. Some of these questions are:

- What is your primary instrument? secondary instruments?
- Did you play any instrument(s) previous to this (these)? If so, how long?
- How long have you been playing this (these) instruments?
- How many hours each week do you perform? practice (solo)? rehearse with others?
- Do you like the music that you play?
- How many years have you played in the above arrangement?
- Location of other instruments/monitors/amplifiers . . . ?
- Do you smoke or is there second-hand smoke in the venue?
- Do you exercise vigorously while performing?
- Are you in good physical shape?
- Do you feel you have any hearing loss?

- Do you have any tinnitus or ringing in your ears?/ nature of the tinnitus?
- Have you had any previous hearing tests?/results?
- Do you have any other problems or concerns or questions relating to your hearing?

The last question generally can involve queries surrounding the psychophysics of hearing and the exact mechanism of future hearing loss. Although this is not an aspect of the case history, the education of the musician typically starts at this point. Full answers to questions about equal loudness contours, a need to equalize, and "testing hearing up to 20,000 Hz" are best left until after the audiometry.

AUDIOMETRIC ASSESSMENT

A full hearing assessment including pure tone, immittance, otoacoustic emission, and speech audiometry is recommended in order to rule out any nonmusic, medically related concerns. Once this is done, the audiogram becomes a teaching tool.

From various studies (Chasin & Chong, 1991, 1992, 1995; Doswell-Royster, Royster, & Killion, 1991), the majority of musicians tested do have an audiometric notch in the 3000–6000 Hz region; thus, an assessment that merely tells us this may be of limited value. The one great diagnostic value of the audiogram, barring other medical etiologies, is that the degree of the "noise/music" notch can yield information regarding an individual's susceptibility to noise/music exposure. That is, a 50 dB HL music notch in the audiogram of a 13-year-old musician may indicate an abnormal susceptibility to exposure. Counseling and follow-up should reflect this. It may also be an indicator of another etiology such as a congenital and/or progressive loss and this should certainly be investigated by the appropriate medical personnel.

As discussed in Chapter 2, damage risk criteria are not well defined for musicians, partly because of the wide ranges of intensities, time periods, and spectra to which musicians are typically exposed. Therefore, we cannot definitively at this point say that a certain degree of hearing loss is statistically out of the norm for such a group and such an age. At most, we typically compare a certain audiometric result with other results we see clinically and make a clinical judgment as to whether the loss *seems* to be excessive. Audiometry, therefore, does have certain limitations in our counseling and clinical mangement.

In explaining the results of audiometry to the musician, it is useful to provide both a conservative and a radical interpretation. The conservative interpretation may be that "this is only a slight hearing loss given your 28 years in the orchestra, so nothing needs to be done. The only thing that has changed is that you have had a hearing test and you know that you have a slight hearing loss." The more radical approach is "what can we do today to ensure that you can still play and enjoy your music in 20 years." Depending on which interpretation is taken, action may or may not be indicated. The exact degree of the hearing loss, the type of music that the musician plays, the instrument category, and the desires of the musician all affect the description of the audiometric results to the musician.

Decreasing audiometric step size or increasing the range of testing to the realm of high-frequency audiometry probably would not increase accuracy and thereby improve counseling. In the absence of damage risk criteria, tightening up accuracy to an ill-defined target would be clinically wasteful. However, given the importance of the audiogram for counseling, the use of otoacoustic emissions which assess the status of the outer hair cells (Lonsbury-Martin & Martin, 1990b; Lonsbury-Martin et al., 1993) may be quite useful. Abnormal results in an otoacoustic emission test may show up prior to an audiometric loss, using conventional techniques, and if the goal is to educate the musician about the potential for future hearing loss, such a testing protocol is feasible (Attias et al., 1995; Hall & Santucci, 1995). A case of abnormal otoacoustic emissions with a normal audiogram is shown in Figure 6–2a. This is contrasted with normal emissions (and a normal audiogram) shown in Figure 6–2b.

SPECTRAL ASSESSMENT OF THE MUSICIAN'S INSTRUMENT

Certain musical instruments are notorious for generating a high noise level that would be far in excess of even the most conservative noise regulations. Recall, however, that most damage risk contours and noise regulations were established for steady state noise, and these musical instruments produce nonsteady state energy outputs. These include percussion, small strings (violin and viola), treble brass (trumpets and French horns), some woodwinds (flute and piccolo), and most amplified instruments. Nevertheless, depending on how they are played, as well as the physical makeup of the component parts (bows, reeds, mouthpieces), the level generated can vary widely. A clinically efficient technique is required that can assess the spectral output in situ. Such a technique was set out by Chasin and Chong (1992) and is described here.

The technique involves the modification of a clinical real ear measurement (REM) system. In this sense, almost any audiological clinical facility has the capability to perform these analyses. REM systems are designed to assess the output of a hearing aid in an individual's ear canal and have been in clinical use since 1983.

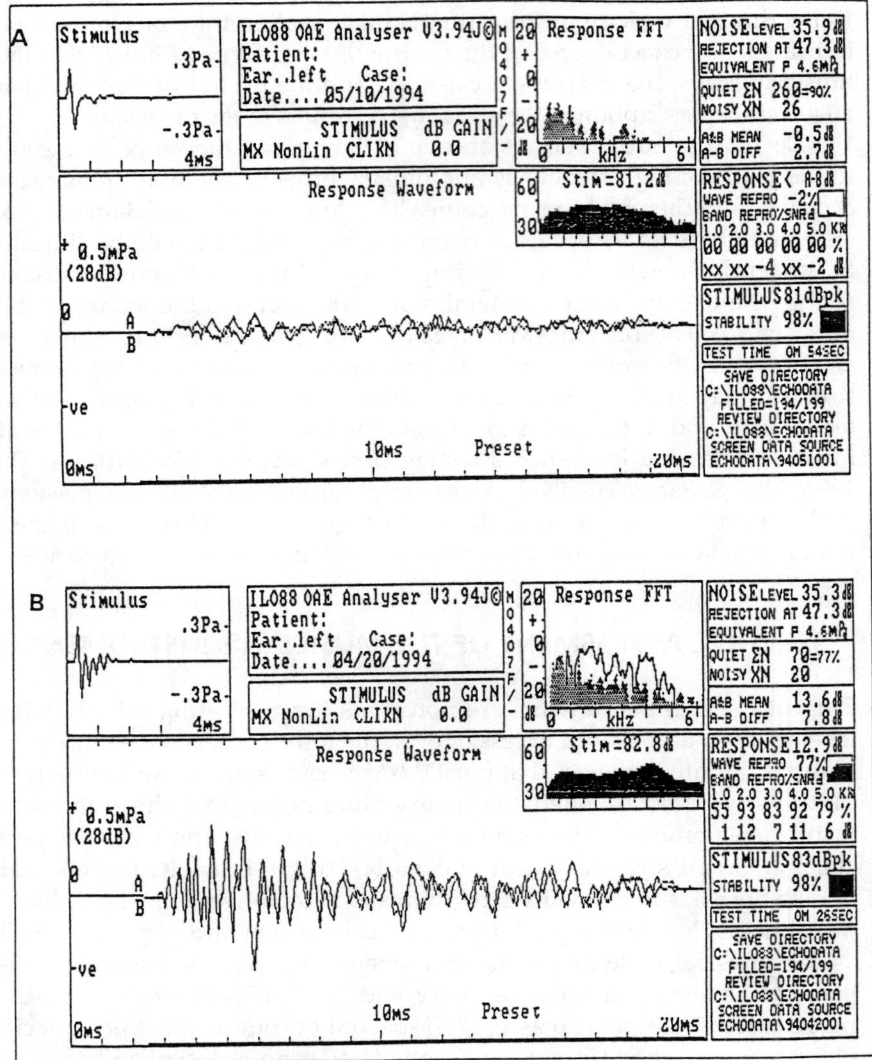

Figure 6–2. Despite both musicians having normal pure-tone audiograms, one musician has abnormal otoacoustic emissions (A) and the other has normal otoacoustic emissions (B). (Courtesy of James Hall, III.)

Two microphones are typically utilized: a test microphone connected to a probe tube that is inserted into the individual's ear canal and a reference microphone situated on the outer portion of the head to monitor the sound level at the point of the hearing aid input. Once calibrated in the normal fashion, the REM system is modified by disabling the reference microphone and disabling the speaker. The REM system now becomes an in situ spectrum analyzer utilizing the test probe tube microphone. The probe tube can then be inserted into the ear canal and placed near the ear drum or be situated in the sound field, depending on the requirements.

Various manufacturers have differing nomenclature for this modification, but terms such as "substitution" (vs. pressure), "reference microphone off" (vs. "on") are used. The owner's manual of the REM device in question should be able to provide information about the appropriate modification. Disabling the speaker may be as simple as physically disconnecting one or both speaker terminals or setting the stimulus level to "off" or "0 dB." Again, the appropriate owner's manual should provide the details.

To obtain estimates of the sound levels and spectral shape that reach a musician's ear, placing the probe tube microphone near the ear drum is sufficient. However, if one desires to obtain an exact spectrum, a sound field measure may be more appropriate. For example, Benade (1990) argues that the most optimal location to measure a single note from a woodwind instrument would be to measure the output with the microphone at the opening of the first noncovered finger hole.

The musician is asked to play and sustain a low-range (frequency) note, a mid-range note, and a note near the upper limits of the instrument in question. The notes must be sustained long enough to allow the modified REM system to perform either a spectral sweep or other digital technique. Each of these three notes is played at a quiet (piano), a medium (mezzo forte) and a loud (forte), level. In this way, the range of intensities and frequencies that this musician plays can be determined. This may differ if the musician uses various bows, reeds, or mouth pieces. Figure 6–3 shows such a spectral analysis performed on one note and at three different playing intensities.

It is important to use the musicians' own terminology at this point since their playing styles and techniques are based on the musical intensity terms of "piano" ranging up to "forte." As we saw in Chapter 1, there is a wide range of variability among these terms as used by different musicians. In addition, since musicians are familiar with the notes of music (A, A#, B, . . .) and audiologists are familiar with frequencies (440 Hz, 466 Hz, . . .), it is useful to use the chart from Appendix I to translate the spectral data on the REM system to equivalent notes.

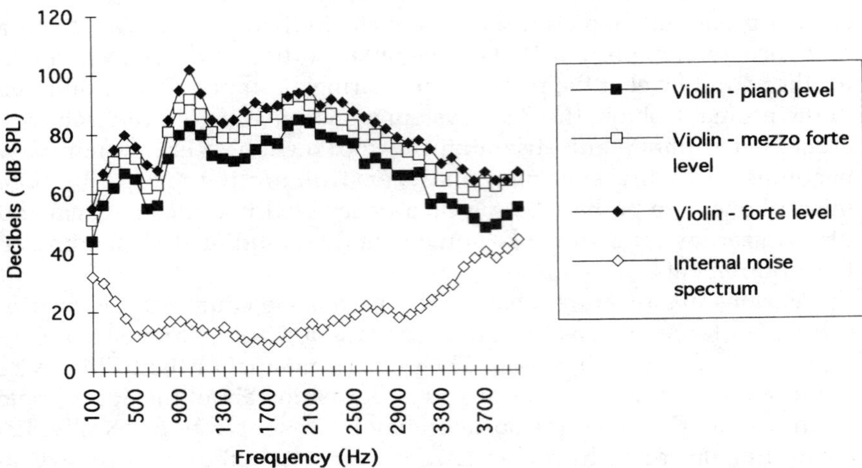

Figure 6–3. Spectral analysis by the modified REM system of a note played at three different levels. Also shown is the internal noise spectrum of the REM system.

The accuracy of such an analysis will depend on several factors (e.g., the number of samples per octave analyzed, the bandwidths of the analyzing filters, and the various time constants of the digital technique such as a Fast Fourier Transform, FFT) that may have been used. The bandwidths of musical notes and their spectral slopes are broader than the analyzing parameters that the modified REM systems typically use, so no major loss (or erroneous aquisition) of information will be observed. The accuracy of the exact center frequency of the note being assessed may be poor due to the bandwidth of the analyzing filters, but this technique is not intended to tune an instrument; it is merely to analyze its salient features.

A factor that can limit the validity of such an analysis is the level of internal noise in the REM system. Newby (1990) pointed out a simple technique to determine the noise floor of a REM system. Once the device is calibrated in the usual fashion according to the procedure set out in the owner's manual, a spectral sweep or other digital technique is performed with the probe tube blocked. The internal noise is displayed (as in Figure 6–3) on the output screen.

Spectral levels at least 10 dB greater than the noise floor are required to ensure that the signal is actually being assessed. If this is not the case, the spectral data are suspect. For all intents and purposes, with modern equipment the only area of real concern is in the higher frequencies (above 4000 Hz).

Other spectral analysis techniques may be utilized, especially for musical instruments that do not generate a steady state note. Guitars, percussion, and piano are examples of instruments that cannot be easily analyzed using this technique. Spectral analysis software programs (such as Signalyze™) are commercially available, many of which can be implemented on laptop computers (with built-in analog-to-digital and digital-to-analog conversion cards) and these prove invaluable, as long as the spectra are measured in the sound field and not in the ear canal.

SPECIFICATION OF REMEDIAL ACTION

The fourth aspect of a musician's assessment involves the recommendations and specification of remedial action, if any. Chapter 5 is dedicated to ear protection and other alternatives and Chapters 7 and 8 cover the specification of many environmental techniques and strategies that can be used to reduce music exposure. The specification for ear protection may be a uniform attenuator earplug such as the ER-15 or ER-25, a frequency-specific one such as the vented/tuned earplug, or a modification of any of the above. Other measures to reduce the potential for further hearing loss may include an intentional use of the stapedius reflex, use of long hair, or an environmental change. Alternative feedback schemes could be implemented in the performance hall to improve the monitoring of one's playing at a significantly lower intensity level.

It may be that as a result of audiologic detective work, one is able to determine that the source(s) of music exposure are no longer present and therefore no changes are required, or it may mean that due to a possibly high level of susceptibility to music exposure, the musician should consider another career. While this last one is extremely rare, it does happen and the "politics" of music and possible compensation and/or retraining comes into play. Chapter 9 is dedicated to this important issue.

VERIFICATION OF THE ATTENUATION CHARACTERISTICS

Like hearing aids, the attenuation characteristics of the specified ear protection should be verified. Three general methods currently exist: (a) insertion loss, (b) real-ear attenuation at threshold (REAT) under headphones, and (c) real-ear attenuation at threshold (REAT) in the sound field. Typically only the first two are clinically utilized. The REAT in the sound field is not typically used because musician ear plugs tend to be quite small, such that an "under the earphone" approach is adequate without concern for sound field ambient noise levels.

Insertion Loss

As discussed in Chapter 5, insertion loss is related to insertion gain and is the difference between the sound pressure level generated in the ear canal with the hearing protector in place and that in the unoccluded ear canal. A probe tube is inserted through a small hole in the hearing protector, whose most medial portion extends at least 4–5 millimeters (mm) beyond the tip of the earplug. The sound pressure level is also measured in the exact same position in the unoccluded ear canal to develop a difference measure—namely, insertion loss. Since an insertion loss measure is a difference measure, there are no units to the resulting decibel figure, just as hearing aid gain is also merely in decibels (and not dB HL or dB SPL, etc.). An excellent review of this and related procedures can be found in Berger (1986).

Caution must be taken to ensure that the probe tube terminates at least 4–5 mm beyond the tip of the hearing protector to avoid obtaining an artifact due to a phenomenon called *spreading inertance*. This high-frequency artifact yields invalid results due to the behavior of incident radial waves interacting with reflected planar waves in the region adjacent to the end of a sound bore. More information can be found on this topic in Chasin (1989b). Another source of error occurs if the measured insertion loss is not at least 10 dB above the noise floor of the REM device.

A modification of this test is to place the probe tube between the ear canal wall and the hearing protector. This should not cause problems unless there is an inadvertant slit leak created, which will compromise the measurement of the attenuation characteristics in the lower frequencies. A sealing substance (e.g., Vaseline) can be used to prevent any leaks. Recently, a new type of probe tube has been developed with a flat exterior that can minimize these problems.

Real-Ear Attenuation at Threshold (REAT)

The REAT of earplugs can also be assessed, which is analogous to functional gain measures with hearing aids. Under audiometric headphones, the difference between the person's threshold is measured in both an unoccluded and occluded situation. Unlike the insertion loss method, a subject must provide a response with an associated variability. If the chosen step size is 5 dB, then such a pair of responses will have a standard error of $\sqrt{(5^2 + 5^2)} = 7$ dB. Choice of a 2 dB step size would reduce the standard error to 2.8 dB. Conventional step sizes in this procedure may then be too large to verify performance reliably, just as functional gain can be a much weaker tool than insertion gain in the assessment of hearing aids.

In addition, if this technique is to be used, the effect of the presence of the earplug under the earphone must be calculated. The presence of the earplug would effectively decrease the volume under the audiometric earphones, thus increasing the generated sound pressure level. This volume-associated change should then be added to the final calculation. To accomplish this, the output of the earphone should first be measured with the modified REM system with the probe tube microphone in the unoccluded condition, and again with the earplug in place with the probe tube sitting in the concha just medial to the earphone in both cases. Such a correction only needs to be performed once and then can be added to the calibration for all similar sized earplugs. Typically, such a decrease in volume only elevates the measured sound pressure level by no more than 1–2 decibels (Chasin, 1994).

VERIFICATION OF THE DEGREE OF OCCLUSION EFFECT

Another aspect of ear protection that needs to be verified is the degree of the occlusion effect. The *occlusion effect* is related to the generation of low-frequency sound energy in the ear canal when the ear canal is occluded. Clinically, comments are made relating to patients hearing their own voices as being too loud or hearing their own breathing. Acoustically, the occlusion effect derives from low-frequency energy in the vocal tract being transduced through the cartilaginous portion of the ear canal wall. If the ear canal is not occluded, this low-frequency energy escapes laterally out of the ear canal and we are not aware of it.

In English (and most languages of the world) the two sounds that yield the greatest occlusion effect are the two high vowels, [i] as in "petite" and [u] as in "lute." Because of the laws governing the acoustic behavior of Helmholtz resonances, these high vowels possess very low-frequency first resonances (or formants). Typically, these vocal-tract induced resonances occur at about 125–150 Hz. And it is this low-frequency energy that is transduced to the ear canal. One can plug the ears and hear a significant increase in the loudness of the vowels [i] and [u], but the same cannot be observed by low vowels such as [a] as in "father."

The modified REM system approach described above can be used to measure the extent of the occlusion effect objectively. The musician should be instructed to say and sustain the vowel [i] while the probe tube is placed in the ear canal with the ear plug in place. The REM system will generate a curve which can be in excess of 20 dB greater than the unoccluded condition at 250 Hz. An earplug that has a minimal occlusion effect will generate less than a 5-decibel greater sound pressure level than in the unoccluded situation. Figure 6–4 shows such a measurement of the occlusion effect for the vowel [i]. Note that this effect is only observed in the lower frequency region.

If a significant occlusion effect does occur, the bore length of the earplug can be extended into the bony portion of the ear canal, upon a

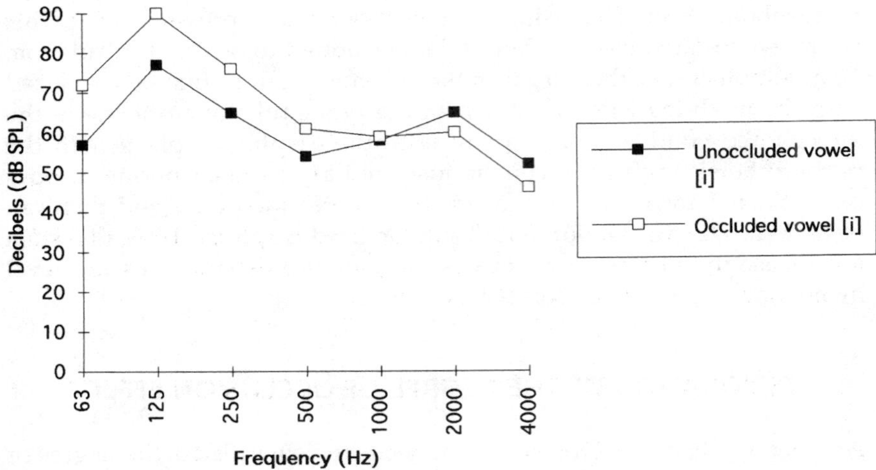

Figure 6–4. Measurement of the occlusion effect on the vowel [i] (as in "petite").

remake. If a musician has a history of problems with the occlusion effect, an ear mold impression can be taken with a deep bore, and the mouth should be held in the [i] position during the curing phase of the impression procedure. That is, have the musician make the mouth position of "eeeee" for at least the first 2 minutes of the impression-taking procedure.

Other than the comfort concern, another reason for minimizing the occlusion effect is that for vocalists, the energy of their lower frequency notes may be enhanced with a poorly made earplug and they may be better off with no ear protection at all.

In a busy clinic, the REM system may be required for other work, so an inexpensive alternative is available that tests and displays the degree of the occlusion effect in decibels at 200 Hz, using the same technology as conventional REM systems.

FOUR EXAMPLES

The following four scenarios illustrate how the methods presented in this chapter can be used for different musicians.

Classical Violinist

A 28-year-old classical violinist is a section player at a local orchestra. She reports mild tinnitus bilaterally, especially when it is quiet, but it is not bothersome. There are no other medical concerns and she does not smoke. The only report of family hearing loss is an elderly uncle who worked in a noisy factory before retiring. She practices alone 2–3 hours each day and gives six weekly performances of 2 hours each. In addition, she has a 2-hour orchestral rehearsal once each week, and she teaches one student for 1 hour, twice each week. Being a section player, she is surrounded by violinists on all sides and sits under an orchestral overhang in a performance pit. She did report that she felt she had to play louder while in the pit than in other locations.

Audiometric testing indicated normal middle ear function bilaterally with a 25 dB audiometric notch in the left ear at 6000 Hz. The right ear had a 15 dB notch at the same frequency.

A spectral assessment with her bow and violin indicated that, at a mezzo forte level, for all notes tested she was obtaining levels in excess of 95 dB SPL for the harmonics even though the fundamental energies were on the order of only 80 dB SPL. Figure 6–5 shows the results of the spectral assessment performed at her left eardrum during a sustained mezzo forte A_4 (440 Hz), with the top curve being before any action is taken. Note that the higher frequency harmonic energy is more intense than the fundamental energy at 440 Hz characteristic of treble instruments.

Broadband ER-15 earplugs were made that uniformly attenuated all sound energy by about 15 decibels. Her violin spectrum with the ER-15 earplugs in place was now approximately 15 decibels less intense and is shown as the bottom curve in Figure 6–5.

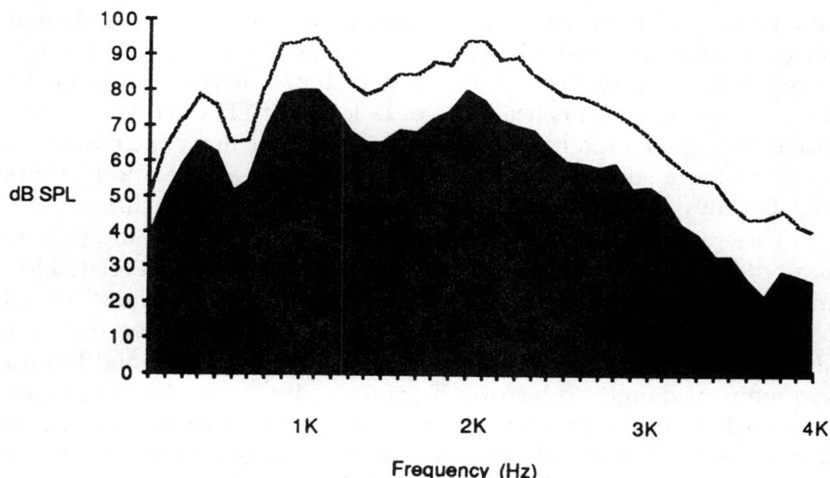

Figure 6–5. Spectrum of a violin playing A_4 (440 Hz) without (top) and with the ER-15 earplug (bottom/black). (From "A Clinically Efficient Hearing Protection Program for Musicians," by M. Chasin & J. Chong, 1992, *Medical Problems of Performing Artists, 7*, p. 42. Copyright 1992 by Hanley & Belfus, Inc. Reprinted with permission.)

In addition, she was moved out from under the orchestral overhang in the pit. The higher frequency harmonics were being attenuated by the presence of the overhang. To compensate for the loss of monitoring caused by the overhang, she was playing harder, which generated a greater overall level. Moving her out from under the overhang reduced her playing level by 2–3 decibels. Both of these alterations—one being ear protection and one being environmental—reduced the overall level at her ear by 17–18 decibels. She was encouraged to wear the ER-15 while practicing and during rehearsals as well as while performing.

Rock and Roll Percussionist

A 25-year-old drummer with a rock group was seen. He had been playing since age 14 and he drums anywhere from 1 hour each month to 18 hours each week. He had no hearing complaints but read in the popular press that drummers should be wearing earplugs. He has been wearing the foam industrial-type earplugs for six months and now desires custom made earplugs. He is right handed and a heavy smoker. There was no reported history of hearing loss in his family. He volunteered that he does have occasional wrist problems especially after a long set. He also reported that he attends noisy night clubs quite often.

Audiometric testing indicated that he has a 35 dB notch at 6000 Hz in his left ear and a 15 dB notch in the right ear. There is normal middle ear function bilaterally.

A spectral assessment could not be performed because of the impulsive nature of his instrument. The technique outlined in this chapter is for only those sources that can maintain a steady signal long enough to perform a sweep or FFT by the REM system. However, a sound level meter was held near his head and peak levels of 122 dBA were obtained while hitting the high hat. Other spectral analysis devices could be used for percussive sounds (such as those implemented on laptop computers), but they are not routinely available in audiological facilities.

The audiometric asymmetry (left ear being worse) suggests that most of his hearing damage derives from his own drum kit related to the high hat cymbals on the left side, as well as from "rim shots" with his left hand. A smaller amount of hearing loss would derive from night clubs. Night clubs, because of the level of reverberation, tend to pose a symmetrical danger to hearing. Because of his wide playing ranges (1 hour each month to 18 hours each week), it is impossible to determine if this loss is consistent with any damage risk criteria for industrial noise.

The ER-25 earplugs were recommended that provide approximately 25 decibels of attenuation up to 6000 Hz. With peak intensity levels in excess of 120 dBA, the milder ER-15 earplugs would not be sufficient. In addition, the foam industrial-strength earplugs were providing excessive attenuations of 35–38 dB. The monitoring of his drum strokes was negatively influenced by this loss of monitoring ability.

With the foam plugs, he hit a practice pad at 113 dBA. Without earplugs, he hit the pad at 103 dBA. With the ER-25 earplugs in place, he hit the practice pad at 104 dB. His EMG (electromyographic) activity also returned to a normal level and complaints of wrist pain ceased. He was counseled regarding the increased propensity he may have for hearing loss because of his heavy smoking, and the role of carbon monoxide in cochlear function was discussed. It was also suggested that he consider altering the style of hitting the high hats on the left side. Some drummers allow the high hat cymbals to close when hitting with a drum stick, as there is less overall intensity than if they are hit while apart. A closed technique would be less damaging than an open one.

Cellist

A 32-year-old cellist was seen for a musician's assessment because of an annoying trumpet behind him. Repeated requests to the conductor and stage manager to move him or the trumpet section were ignored. When the trumpet player was asked to move his music stand, he just laughed. There is no reported hearing loss and no tinnitus. There is no reported family history of hearing loss. He practices 3 hours each day and performs 8 shows each week in a Broadway-type production. There are no regular rehearsals.

Audiometric testing indicated normal hearing in both ears. Otoacoustic emissions were not assessed.

A spectral assessment of his cello indicated that at a mezzo forte level, he was only able to generate a peak of 82 dB SPL at his left ear. At a forte level he was able to obtain a peak level of 86 dB SPL. Clearly, he is not in danger of hearing impairment from his own instrument, but the trumpet section to his rear may pose a different situation. Other than the reported annoyance from this source, there is the real danger of future hearing loss from the trumpet section.

On behalf of the musician, the clinic staff arranged a discussion with the stage manager and head of the local musician's union. Typical of many shows of this type, there was initial resistance until it was pointed out that adjustments would not be excessively expensive and would probably improve the quality of the music. The staff recommended that the trumpet section be put on risers, since the damaging higher frequency harmonic energy of the trumpet is highly directional. Placing the section on risers meant that much of the damaging and annoying music energy would literally go over the heads of those musicians who were "downstream." (For more information on this phenomenon see Chapters 4 and 8.)

In addition, a pair of vented/tuned earplugs were made which provided significant attenuation to only those sounds above 2000 Hz. All of the musically relevant energy of the cello was left unaffected, but extraneous higher frequency harmonic energy from other sources was reduced.

Ex-Rock and Roll Guitarist

A 47-year-old electric guitar player who now only plays "relatively quiet pop" music in a solo environment was seen for a musician's assessment. His primary complaint was that he could not hear the "top end of the sound." He is gainfully employed in a nonmusical career and only plays his guitar on occasional weekends. Although he has never had his hearing tested, he is sure that he has a hearing loss and doesn't want to lose anymore. He has no other reported medical problems.

Audiometric testing indicated a bilateral high-frequency loss consistent with presbycusis and noise/music exposure. His loss is such that a mild high-frequency emphasis hearing aid is certainly a possibility.

His "relatively quiet pop" music was assessed with a sound level meter at the level of his ear and found to be approximately 87 dBA.

One approach would be to do nothing since he is out of a high music environment and only plays on occasion. An hour or two at 87 dBA each month should pose no threat to his hearing.

However, he is concerned enough—even after being told that nothing really needs to be done—to want to obtain some earplugs. Although the optimal recommendation would be for a pair of ER-15 earplugs, a drawback is that the slight 15 dB decrease in the higher frequencies (in addition to his sensorineural hearing loss) may be sufficient to cause him to lose even more of the "top end of the sound." A modification is therefore possible to the ER-15. As discussed in Chapter 5, a pair of ER-15 earplugs with a longer and a narrower bore than is typical will cause less attenuation in the 4000 Hz region. The modified ER-15 will then function as an attenuator for the lower and mid frequencies but with only a very slight attenuation for the 4000 Hz region.

As an alternative, a mild gain level-dependent hearing aid (such as a K-AMP™) with an input limiter set very high such that there is no clipping of the input music would also be useful (L. Revit, personal communication, 1995). Figure 6–6 shows an input/output curve for one such hearing aid. Because of the level-dependent character of the hearing aid, there is attenuation for high input levels.

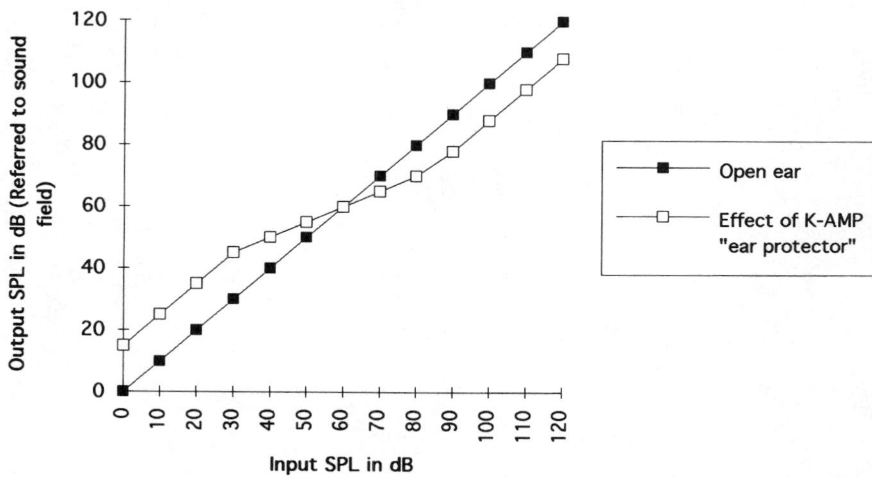

Figure 6–6. Input/output curve for a hearing aid with a K-AMP™ circuit functioning as an electronic attenuator. While there is 15 dB of low-level gain, there is 12 dB of high-level attenuation. (Adapted by permission of Etymotic Research.)

SUMMARY

Audiometric testing of the musician is only a small part of the clinical assessment. Of greater importance is the spectral assessment (or the knowledge) of the musical instrument and the specification of remedial action. Other than the recommendation of hearing protectors (Chapter 5), much of the remedial action will be discussed further in Chapters 7 and 8.

The assessment begins with an extended (and forensic) case history so that all sources of noise and music exposure can be evaluated. Risk factors, such as smoking, can be identified and appropriate counseling given.

A modified REM system is used to assess the acoustic output of the musical instrument that takes into account individual factors, such as playing style and instrument quality. For instruments where a sustained note cannot be made for proper analysis (such as percussion), commercially available "speech spectral analysis" software programs can be quite useful.

Verification of the attenuation characteristics and the occlusion effect of the specified hearing protectors can be accomplished with an insertion loss measure or by a subjective threshold based approach (REAT). Other measures are available, but tend to lack the test–retest reliability of the insertion loss and REAT techniques.

SUMMARY

CHAPTER

7

Room Acoustics

INTRODUCTION

This chapter will equip the audiologist with information to answer some basic questions regarding the acoustics of performance halls. These venues may range from dedicated concert halls and renovated churches to small restaurants and school gymnasiums.

Since the time of Wallace Sabine, who was considered the father of modern architectural acoustics (Beranek, 1992), four essential features of a good performance hall have been delineated. These are (1) an adequately intense sound level (both for the listener and the musician), (2) an early first sound reflection, (3) sound that is evenly distributed, and (4) reverberation characteristics that are appropriate for the type of music being played.

Adequately Intense Sound Level

Many performance halls have had several of these four essential features, but even the best have not had all in perfect balance. For example, the early Greek amphitheaters, although known for their excellent acoustics, had relatively low sound levels if measured at a significant

---

Bill Gastmeier, M.A.S.c., P.Eng., has co-written this chapter in order to provide an applied orientation to what would otherwise be a purely academic overview. Mr. Gastmeier is a consulting engineer in acoustics, noise, and vibration.

distance from the performer (Campbell & Greated, 1987). The ancient Greeks certainly could have benefited from an electrical amplification system to supplement the sound levels for those in the "inexpensive seats." In modern performance halls, there are two frequently utilized techniques for enhancing the sound level: through the use of reflective surfaces (baffles) and the use of electrical amplification/monitoring systems. Electrical systems will be discussed in more detail later in this chapter.

"Clouds" have been utilized to enhance the sound levels near the rear of many performance halls. Clouds are reflective baffles suspended above many classical orchestras and are angled in such a way as to provide a directed reflection toward the rear of the performance hall. The angle is determined by the application of geometric or "ray acoustics" where the analogy is drawn with optics (light and mirrors). As the angle of incidence is always equal to the angle of reflection, the tilt of each surface can be selected to provide even coverage for all of the seating area. The clouds must be quite large and rigid to provide significant reflections, particularly at lower frequencies. To be effective at reflecting the deep basstones, they must also be fairly massive.

A useful characterstic of these baffles is that their orientation and height can be altered depending on the performance hall and type of music. They can be adjusted lower for many types of modern music and raised for organ and Romantic music. In some cases, a movable orchestra "shell" can be created within the stage house of a proscenium theater, projecting sound to the audience instead of allowing it to be absorbed by the stage house.

Early First Sound Reflections

Rarely does an acoustic technique have just one function. Suspended acoustic baffles, such as clouds, can also serve to provide an early first sound reflection. Figure 7–1 shows the direct sound followed by the first reflection off the walls, and/or ceilings. Subsequent reflections come later and merge into a reverberation pattern that characterizes a hall.

The work of Beranek (1962), Ando and Gottlob (1979), and others has indicated that if the first reflection is less than 20–22 msec after the initial direct sound, then there is a feeling of "intimacy." It is generally the best if these first reflections emanate from the lateral walls of the performance hall (Marshall, 1967, 1968). Hidaka, Beranek, and Okano (1995) referred to this measure as the initial-time-delay gap and noted that for near-rectangular halls, it can be calculated from architectural blueprints. Barron and Marshall (1981) noted that, in general, as the number of early lateral reflections increased, the music gained "body" and "fullness."

Beranek (1962) felt that the best halls should have at least five equally spaced reflections in the first 60 msec after the initial sound and that this contributed to the "texture" of the music.

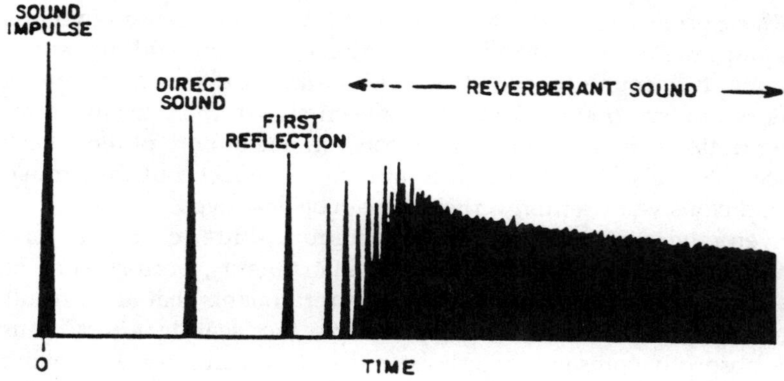

Figure 7–1. Multiple reflections of a sound impulse as heard by a listener. (From *The Acoustical Foundations of Music* [p. 165] by J. Backus, 1977, New York: W. W. Norton & Company, Inc. Copyright 1977 by W. W. Norton & Company, Inc. Reprinted with permission.)

However, since sound traverses a distance of approximately 7 m in 20 msec, listeners who sit further than 7 m from a wall would not feel as intimate as those who sit nearer the walls. This is understandably a more significant problem for larger theaters.

The clouds that are suspended above the orchestra can be utilized to effectively alter the time of the first reflection, thus improving the sensation of intimacy. Other acoustic baffles and reflectors can be utilized elsewhere in performance halls to alter the initial-time-delay gap as well as to improve the uniformity of the sound field in the room. For example, coverings or other baffle structures may be necessary in churches with domes or high vaulted ceilings into order to diffuse this type of ceiling's natural sound focusing ability.

Evenly Distributed Sound

Parallel surfaces can be another acoustic defect. Clouds and other sound absorbing or diffusing structures can be set up to alleviate a phenomenon called *flutter echo*. Flutter echo is the audible series of closely spaced echoes that occur when an initial impulse passes repeatedly by the listener. Another defect is the creation of standing waves in a performance hall caused by an incidence and a reflected wave interacting constructively and destructively. Locations in a performance hall can be significantly louder or quieter than others that are just a little distance away, particularly with respect to deep bass tones. Flutter echo can be caused by parallel walls and can even be due to the interaction of the floor and the ceiling. It is commonly encountered when an architecturally old church is converted for more modern music. Clouds have been shown to be useful in minimizing flutter echo. Curtains (with pleats) on one or both of the reflective surfaces have also been used to minimize this effect, but they must be used judiciously or useful reverberance can be destroyed.

Even environments designed to minimize flutter echo may have a nonuniform sound field. Like musical instruments, performance halls have inherent resonants (formants) and antiresonants that are a result of the geometry and room content. For example, the "seat-dip effect," caused by the absorptive presence of upholstered seating, can cause a lessening of energy in the 100–400 Hz region. Judiciously positioned and angled baffles, as well as electrical equalization techniques, can be useful in equalizing a room, in order to negate this low-frequency loss of sound energy.

Reverberation Time

The construction of Boston's Symphony Hall, in 1900, marks the first application of Wallace Sabine's research into a measure called *reverberation time*. Today, the Boston Symphony Hall [along with the Grosser Musikvereinssaal (1870) in Vienna and the Concertgebouw (1887) in Amsterdam] is considered one of the best in existence (Bradely, 1991; Hidaka et al., 1995).

Reverberation time (RT) is the length of time (in seconds) for a sound to decay by 60 decibels. Specifically, RT is proportional to the volume (m^3) of the hall and inversely proportional to the hall's total sound absorption (m^2). Generally, the greater the number of seats (particulary if they are padded), the greater the sound absorption. A large-volume structure with minimal sound absorption such as an underground car garage will have a long RT. In contrast, a library with a high level of sound absorption due to an acoustical tile ceiling, carpeting, and shelves full of books will have a short RT.

It is interesting to note the relationship between the various styles of music and the performance halls of their day. Beranek (1992) noted that baroque music (1600–1750) tended to be played in palace music rooms that were rectangular and full of nonabsorbing ornamentation. RTs were typically between 1.6 and 2.0 seconds and the music was composed accordingly. Such a long RT allows the listener to hear each note as being "prolonged and the music takes on a singing tone" (Beranek, 1992, p. 2). The Romantic period of music of the late nineteenth century and the early twentieth century was written for halls with even longer RTs. Kuhl (1954, cited in Beranek, 1992) performed a series of experiments using artificially created reverberations and found that RTs of approximately 1.5 seconds were desired for classical music, and RTs of 2.0 seconds were desired for music of the Romantic period.

Table 7–1 shows desired RTs for the mid frequencies for a wide selection of activities. The values in Table 7–1 are only approximate because of the uncontrolled factor of room volume. These figures, however, are for typical room sizes associated with the type of music.

Table 7–1 shows several interesting characteristics. Long RTs, such as those found in organ music, tend to facilitate the "ringing" and sound enhancement that is an essential part of this music. Most modern facilities such as the Boston Symphony Hall (1.85 seconds) tend to have RTs in the 1.7–2.0 category. Longer RTs tend to degrade speech clarity and as can be observed, speech conference rooms tend to have RTs of less than 1.0 seconds. However, most musicians find that performance halls with RTs as short as 1.0 second tend to be "dead" and hard to play in. It may be difficult to hear their colleagues and the lack of reverberance makes the sound dull and lifeless.

The data from Table 7–1 indicate clearly that a multipurpose hall (i.e., one that is used for speech as well as music) can be very difficult to construct, unless changeable acoustic baffling and/or an electronic mechanism is in place to alter the RT (Bradley, 1991).

Table 7–2 shows that a superior, a good, and a fair-to-good concert hall can have similar RTs, despite the dramatic difference in subjective preference. The single measure of RT cannot in itself account for the subjective quality preference of a performance hall. Following is a discussion of some other measures that may be a better indicator than RT.

More Complex Reverberation Measures

The C_{80} ratio of early to late sound energy is determined by the energy summed in the first 80 msec as compared to the reflected energy that arrives later (Bradley, 1990). This ratio correlates highly with clarity (temporal definition). Good clarity (a high C_{80}) indicates a high ratio of

Table 7–1. Desired Reverberation Times (RT)

Music Type	RT
Opera	1.3–1.6
Chamber Music	1.0–1.5
Concert Halls	1.7–2.0
Modern Music	1.1–1.7
Organ Music	1.5–2.5
Romantic Music	2.0–2.3
Live Theater	1.0
Speech Conference Rooms	0.4 - 0.9

Table 7–2. Different Quality Concert Halls but Similar Reverberation Times (RT)

Concert Hall	Quality	RT
Boston, Symphony Hall	Superior	1.85
San Francisco, Davies Hall	Good	1.85
London, Barbican Large Hall	Fair-to-Good	1.7

Note: Adapted from Hidaka et al., 1995.

direct sound and early reflections arriving earlier than 80 msec to the remainder of the energy arriving later than 80 msec. A low C_{80} indicates a lack of early reflections and excessive reverberation. One reason for the success and lasting usefulness of rectangular music halls is that strong early reflections are provided by the side walls as well as the ceiling, thereby enhancing clarity.

The interaural cross-correlation coefficient (IACC) is a measure of the difference in sound between the two ears with the listener facing the source (Hidaka et al., 1995). It correlates well with spaciousness since the sensation of spaciousness depends strongly on early lateral (horizontal) reflections.

These measures are now being used to quantify and investigate that special combination of science and art that results in "good acoustics." As reverberation and early arriving reflections are involved in a sometimes contradictory fashion, it is not possible to design a single room that is appropriate for all types of music. Many music performance halls are therefore provided with variable acoustical elements. Retractable curtains are popular as well as more sophistocated variable elements that can be adjusted to expose either reflective or absorptive surfaces. Another scheme to alter the RT is to vary the volume. In some auditoriums, the entire ceiling can be raised or lowered to match the reverberance and patterns of reflected sound energy to the intended funtions. In practice, such spaces are not often fully utilized because of the economic temptation to always use the largest seating capacity.

The use of a sound reinforcement system to increase loudness is discouraged for most classical music performances. In contrast, electronic reverberation enhancement systems have had some success introducing reverberant energy into "dry" spaces (i.e., one with a short RT).

Scale modeling can be utilized in the design of a concert hall since modifications and "fine tuning" can be expensive and embarrassing. Scale modeling is accomplished by using a spark generator located on the stage of a 1/20 model. Makrinenko (1994) has used this method extensively with good results in the Soviet Union. The surface materials are carefully chosen with appropriately defined reflective properties. A microphone is located at various seating positions and the time trace of the initial impulse and resultant reflections is analyzed to determine the significance of various surfaces in providing reflected energy. By covering the surfaces with absorptive materials, defects can be identified.

REHEARSAL ROOMS

Rehearsal rooms are relatively small spaces compared to concert halls. A minimum volume of at least 17 cubic meters per student is necessary or sound levels can be high enough to pose a risk to hearing health (Gastmeier, Pernu, & Chasin, 1994). Successful designs use irregular-shaped rooms with surfaces that provide a balance of diffusion (so players can hear each other) and absorption (to control reverberation and reduce sound levels). Private practice booths should be available that offer low RTs, well-selected acoustical finishes, and a noise-attenuating construction.

SPACES WITH MIXED ACOUSTIC REQUIREMENTS

It is commonplace to hear a visiting baroque group perform at a local church or a pop group in the community hall. The following section is an overview of some of the design parameters of performance venues that have various mixed uses. These venues include (1) worship spaces, (2) theater stages, and (3) community halls. A delineation of the design strengths and/or weaknesses of these multipurpose venues will serve as a basis for the understanding of the limitations of the various forms of music that may be played.

Worship Spaces

As stated earlier, medieval churches, particularly large cathedrals, have excessive reverberation and a resulting lack of speech intelligibility. These factors influenced the style of organ music composed in the period and left their mark on the liturgy. Polyphonic choral music and chanting were developed to take advantage of the extremely long RTs.

Many modern worship spaces are designed to encourage a verbal and musical dialogue between the leader and the congregation. If acoustic conditions are too dry (short RTs), speech may be intelligible, but organ music lacks strength and congregational response is weak.

Some congregations, particularly since the advent of electronic ministry, rely heavily on amplified sound and music, with little congregational participation. These worship spaces require short RTs, taking the form of theaters suitable for radio or television production.

Church buildings may consist of several coupled spaces (e.g., nave, chancel, organ and choir loft). Good design practice indicates that the chancel and pulpit should be well elevated and surrounded with reflective surfaces. The organ and choir should also be in an area surrounded with reflective surfaces. Carpet is avoided and lines of sight between organist, worship leader, choir master, and choir are carefully considered. All background noise sources are controlled and the basic shape of the congregational seating area must be carefully designed for even sound distribution.

With good acoustical design, satisfactory performance can be obtained without a public address system in small and medium sized churches. However, the desire for high ceilings and other architectural features generally results in increasing the volume per seat and a sound reinforcement system may be required even in relatively small churches, particularly for less-audible talkers.

While such high ceiling churches may be appropriate for visiting baroque and Romantic music ensembles, they would be inappropriate for those types of music requiring shorter RTs (see Table 7–1).

Theater Stages

The basic theater stage is the proscenium stage where the performers are in a separate stage house, viewed through a "picture frame." In front of the picture frame are the open and arena stages where the performing area is entirely surrounded by the audience. In open and arena stages, sound-reflecting surfaces such as suspended baffles are extremely important to provide adequate reflected sound.

In the proscenium stage, a sound-reflective orchestra shell is often necessary for a successful musical performance. It projects the sound from the orchestra (in the stage house) into the audience seating area, preventing much of the sound energy from being absorbed in the stage house. Such a shell can be temporarily erected for visiting orchestras to the theater stage venue.

Community Halls

These spaces often exhibit poor acoustics because of hard parallel room surfaces causing flutter echoes and excessive reverberation. Floors are often bare for dancing and cleanability. Ceilings are often made of reflective drywall or plaster and walls are often concrete block for reasons of cost and maintenance. Several things can be done to improve the acoustics of these spaces:

1. An elevated stage should be provided.
2. The ceiling above the stage and at the front of the hall should be reflective.

3. The stage floor should protrude as far as possible into the audience area.
4. Side walls should be broken or splayed to diffuse sound. Absorptive treatments such as cloth-covered fiberglass panels are often used at the rear ceiling and walls of the room.

ELECTRICAL AMPLIFICATION SYSTEMS

To prevent or resolve some problems with many performance halls, electrical amplification systems have been successfully used. In some cases, complicated arrays of speakers and microphones are set up to alter the RT and to ensure sufficient loudness. In some performing environments, an electrical amplification system may be mandatory. For example, while an outdoor concert that uses a bandshell would be heard farther away than one without an acoustic reflector system, an amplication system is still necessary, especially to effectively transmit the lower frequency sounds. As reviewed in Chapter 3, low-frequency sounds, because of their long wavelengths, do not reflect easily, and thus would require an electronic means of transmission. The Greek amphitheaters mentioned earlier would still require electronic amplification to comfortably reach the seats situated higher on the hillside.

Electrical amplification systems have been quite useful for re-establishing a feeling of intimacy in larger performing halls (Bradley, 1991). Well-situated speakers, with appropriate sound delays, can be useful in simulating the optimal acoustics of a much smaller venue. While it is relatively easy to reduce RT by the use of baffles, *assisted resonance* (Parkin, Allen, Purkis, & Scholes, 1953) is an electrical system designed to simulate a longer RT. The Royal Festival Hall in London, England, is a well-known example of this where a series of microphones and speakers (along with 172 pass band filters) were employed to artificially increase the low-frequency RT, after the hall was completed.

Unless modified, electrical amplification systems can create the unfortunate sensation that sound is coming from the loudspeakers rather than from the stage. This phenomenon is called the *precedence effect*, whose characteristics were first delineated by Wallach, Newman, and Rosenzweig (1949). The direction of the first sound wave will define the perceived direction of subsequent sound energy. If a loudspeaker is used and is situated in an audience, the sound from the loudspeaker will be heard before the sound from the stage. This is because electrical energy transduced by the loudspeaker is a faster process (i.e., the speed of electricity) than that emanating from the stage (i.e., the slower speed of sound). However, if the sound from the loudspeaker is artificially delayed 50 msec, listeners will perceive the sound as coming from the stage, despite a higher intensity sound coming from the loudspeakers. Clearly, loudspeakers situated up on the stage would not have this problem.

Pop and rock musical groups that are entirely based on electronic amplification have several advantages over those that are limited by the acoustics of the performance hall. Commercially available electronically controlled equalization and echo/reverberation systems can be used to simulate many different lengths of RT as well as establish any number of early reflections in the performance hall in order to create a sense of intimacy. Ideally, sound engineers for these groups prefer rooms with short RTs, such as those found in speech conference rooms, so that they can create their own RT electronically. However, as discussed in the last section, most pop and rock performance venues are multipurpose halls and tend to be highly reverberant. Little can be done by the sound engineer to ameliorate this.

In many cases, especially in performance halls with undesirable RT characteristics such as those associated with pop and rock music, effective on-stage monitoring of one's own instrument as well as those of the other musicians can be almost impossible. Traditionally, the intensity of the musicians' monitors are increased to an excessive level, and this may in turn cause the musician to play at an inappropriate level. Recently, however, a number of manufacturers have begun to offer in-the-ear earphone monitors. These devices may be custom or noncustom, but essentially negate the requirement of good on-stage monitoring. The earphone monitors are usually coupled to the sound board via a wireless FM route so the musician is free to move, while receiving a well-controlled binaural input. These earphones will be discussed further in Chapter 8.

SUMMARY

The basic assessment measures and remediation techniques, along with their limitations, were reviewed. A good performance hall must have four features: an adequate sound level, an early first sound reflection, evenly distributed sound, and an appropriate reverberation characteristic for the type of music being played.

One commonly used device are clouds. These are reflective baffles that are suspended above many orhcestras and are angled in such a way as to provide a directed reflection toward the rear of the performance hall. They can be adjusted depending on the type of music being played.

The first sound reflection in a hall should be less than 22 msec after the initial direct sound in order for a feeling of intimacy to be established. Both acoustic and electrical techniques are utilized to create this feeling in a large hall that would otherwise not be considered intimate. These techniques also serve to ensure an even distribution of sound.

The RT is a function of both the volume and the absorptive characteristics of the performance hall. An RT that is too long will degrade speech intelligibility and one that is too short will create a feeling of deadness. Different styles of music require different RTs. More complex RT measures, such as the C_{80}, have become quite useful. These measures assess the ratio of early reflections to ones arriving later.

Many good multipurpose facilities that serve as a venue for different styles of music have adjustable acoustic and electrical systems that allow for different RTs. Suggestions are provided for a variety of different environments (worship spaces, theater stages, and community halls) that musicians might find themselves performing in.

CHAPTER

8

Clinical and Environmental Strategies to Reduce Music Exposure

INTRODUCTION

This chapter provides an overview of some clinically expeditious techniques shown to be successful at reducing the potential for music exposure. The techniques are actively in use by many musicians and are felt to be acceptable in a wide range of performing environments. These strategies and techniques are not accepted by all musicians and are typically suggested on a trial-and-error basis. Some of these environmental changes form the basis for the world's first safety guidelines for the Live Performance Industry, established by the Ontario Ministry of Labour in Canada (1993). A "strategy sheet" summaring much of the following information (with relevant figure numbers) can be found in Appendix I and in Table 8–3.

An example of a simple alteration to any performing environment is to place the performing group two meters back from the edge of the stage. This is not always possible to accomplish in practice, especially in the smaller performance halls, but significant high-frequency amplification can result. Musicians would not have to play as vigorously, with the result of a lower overall sound level with potentially less physical and ergonomic strain.

The physics of the high-frequency emphasis shown in Figure 8–1 is related to the wavelength of the sounds (covered in greater detail in Chapter 3). Short wavelength, high-frequency energy acoustically "sees" the floor as an obstruction and thus reflects. In contrast, long wavelength, low-frequency sound energy does not view the floor as a reflective obstruction and is thereby lost to the audience. It should be pointed out that the data in Figure 8–1 is from only one set of measurements (Chasin & Chong, 1995). Such a result is highly variable and depends intimately on the characteristics of the performance hall.

This chapter is organized around seven "musical instrument" categories: (1) small strings, (2) large strings, (3) brass, (4) woodwinds, (5) percussion, (6) amplified instruments, and (7) vocalists.

MUSICAL INSTRUMENT CATEGORIES

Small Stringed Instruments

The instruments in this category include the violins and the violas. As discussed in Chapter 5, the ear protection of choice is the ER-15 earplug, as this will provide broadband uniform attenuation. Sound levels in

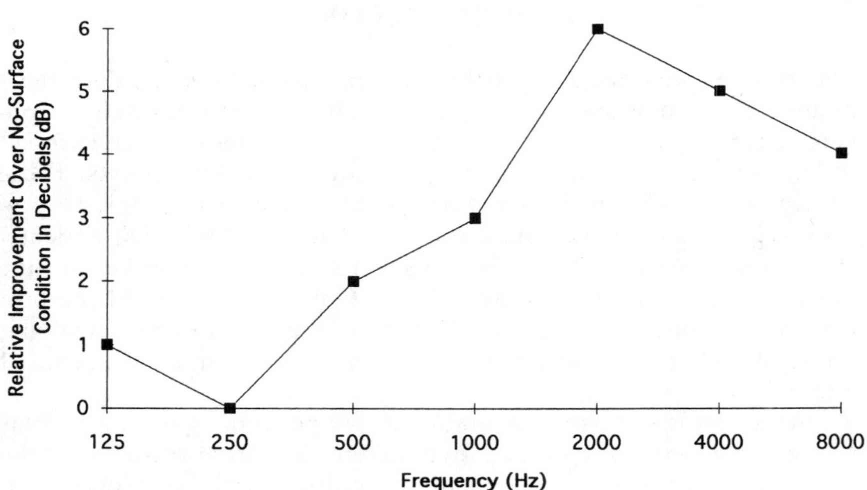

Figure 8–1. High-frequency emphasis that can be achieved by placing the performing group two meters back from the edge of the stage. (From "Four Environmental Techniques to Reduce the Effect of Music Exposure on Hearing," by M. Chasin & J. Chong, 1995, *Medical Problems of Performing Artists, 10,* p. 68. Copyright 1995 by Hanley & Belfus, Inc. Reprinted with permission.)

excess of 110 dB SPL have been measured even when played at an average, or mezzo forte, loudness.

The most important aspect is the positioning of this instrument. Violin and viola players should never be placed under an overhang that is within 1 meter of their heads. Such poorly constructed overhangs for "performance pits" are commonplace at many theater, ballet, and opera performances. Space limitations tend to define the size and dimensions of such performance pits. The higher frequency components of these instruments can be absorbed by the underside of the overhang with the result of a loss of harmonic monitoring. Since the higher frequency harmonic structure is crucial to a perception of proper playing for these instruments, violinists and violists tend to overplay in order to re-establish the correct harmonic balance. Arm and wrist damage can easily result.

Figure 8–2 shows the effect of a poorly constructed overhang on the spectrum of a violin playing A_4 (440 Hz), compared with a spectrum of the same note played in "the open." Loss of some high-frequency harmonic energy would not be a problem for some other instrument categories.

Another useful technique for violins and violas is to use a mute while practicing. Such a mute fits over the bridge of the instrument and attenuates sound energy by adding an extra mass component to the bridge transduction system. Depending on the style of the practice mute, differing degrees of attenuation may be realized.

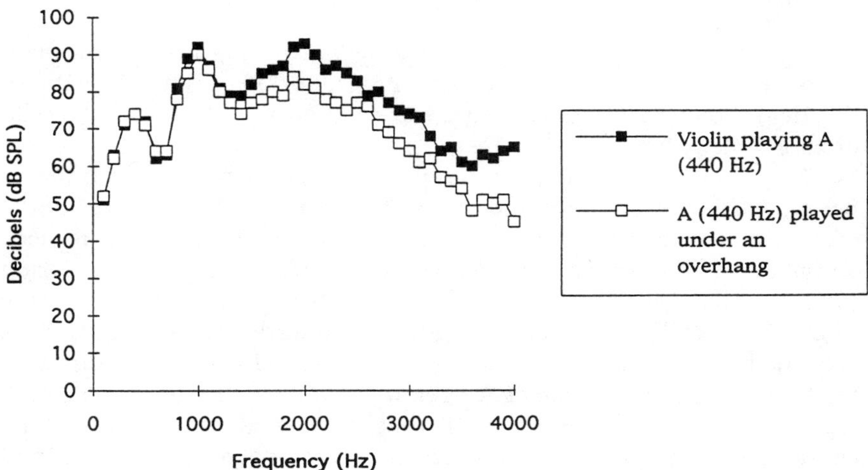

Figure 8–2. Effect on the spectrum of A_4 (440 Hz) of a poorly constructed overhang as compared with no overhang. (From "Four Environmental Techniques to Reduce the Effect of Music Exposure on Hearing," by M. Chasin & J. Chong, 1995, *Medical Problems of Performing Artists, 10*, p. 68. Copyright 1995 by Hanley & Belfus, Inc. Reprinted with permission.)

Large Stringed Instruments

The cello, bass, and harp are the three major instruments in this category. Like all stringed instruments, it is crucial to hear the high-frequency harmonic content; however, because of the larger physical size, most of the important harmonic energy is below 2000 Hz. Placing these musicians under a poorly constructed performance pit overhang will subsequently have little acoustic and ergonomic effect on their playing.

Partly because of the large size of these instruments, the sound levels generated are not excessively great. However, the brass section is typically located to their immediate rear, and it is this source that is the potential threat to hearing loss.

As discussed in Chapter 5, the ear protection of choice is the vented/tuned earplug. This earplug serves to allow most of the fundamental and higher frequency harmonic energy of these instruments through with minimal alteration in the spectrum. However, these earplugs provide a significant high-frequency roll-off in the attenuation pattern. The vented/tuned earplug (typically with a 3 mm inner diameter) can be ideal for the large stringed instruments as it attenuates only the higher frequency sounds of the brass section to their rear.

Belled instruments, such as the trumpet, are highly directional, but only for the higher frequency sounds. This directional characteristic of the trumpet as a function of playing angle was shown in Figure 3–12 (in Chapter 3). If the trumpet section is placed on risers, most of the damaging high-frequency energy literally goes over the heads of the musicians "downwind."

Another strategy successfully used by large string instrument players is an acoustic monitoring device. Figure 8–3 shows a schematic of this device that serves to transduce low-frequency energy from the cello or bass directly to the ear.

Many cello players lean on the pegs of their instrument in order to better hear its low-frequency response that is masked by the rest of the orchestra. This can be inefficient and, in some cases, can lead to neck strain. A 300 mm length (approximately 1 foot) of standard #13 hearing aid tubing that is closed at one end is woven through the strings near the pegs of the cello. A slightly longer tube length can be used for an acoustic bass. This is coupled to the vented/tuned earplug by inserting the tubing directly into the vent opening. Standard #13 hearing aid tubing should fit snugly into the open vent. A male adaptor for the tubing can also be used and can connect directly to either a vented/tuned earplug or an ER-series earplug.

This system characterizes a quarter wavelength resonator with a first mode of resonance at 250–300 Hz. Low-frequency energy is transduced from the strings to the vented/tuned earplug, thus providing improved low-frequency monitoring by up to 11 dB. For other less

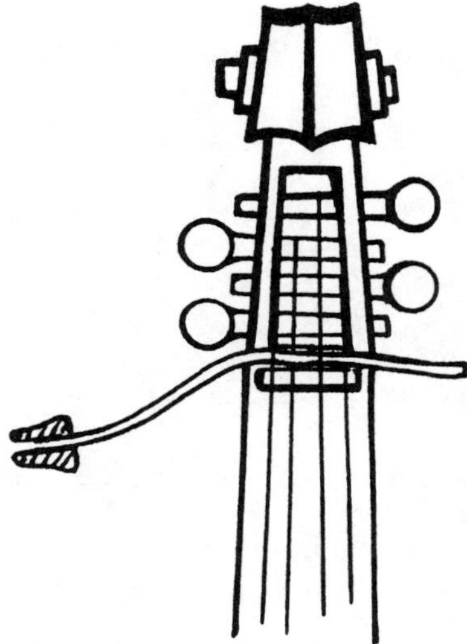

Figure 8–3. Cello acoustic monitoring device that serves to transduce low-frequency energy from the cello or bass, directly to the musician's ear.

"noisy" pieces, the cellist may remove the monitoring tube and use the vented/tuned earplug in the normal fashion. Figure 8–4 shows the low-frequency improvement when the monitoring tube is used.

Brass Instruments

Typical instruments of this category are the trumpet, French horn, trombone, and assorted bass instruments such as the tuba and baritone. Chapter 4 delineated the essential acoustic characteristics of brass instruments. Two important characterstics are that brass instruments are directional for higher frequency energy and that this energy is significantly more intense than the lower frequency fundamental energy. The instrument that can generate the most intense music in this category is the trumpet and for this reason it will be used as the example.

Since trumpet players generate high-frequency spectra that are highly directional (along the playing plane of the instrument), overhangs in performance pits are not a factor. Typically brass sections are placed to the rear of an orchestra or band because of their high intensity and it is this location that is frequently covered by an overhang.

It is recommended, however, that whenever possible, the trumpet section should be on risers, as this will allow the higher frequency intense harmonic energy to go over the head of the musicians in front of them. The data in Table 8–1 were measured at the position of the cellist, approximately 1.5 meters in front of the trumpet player. The difference

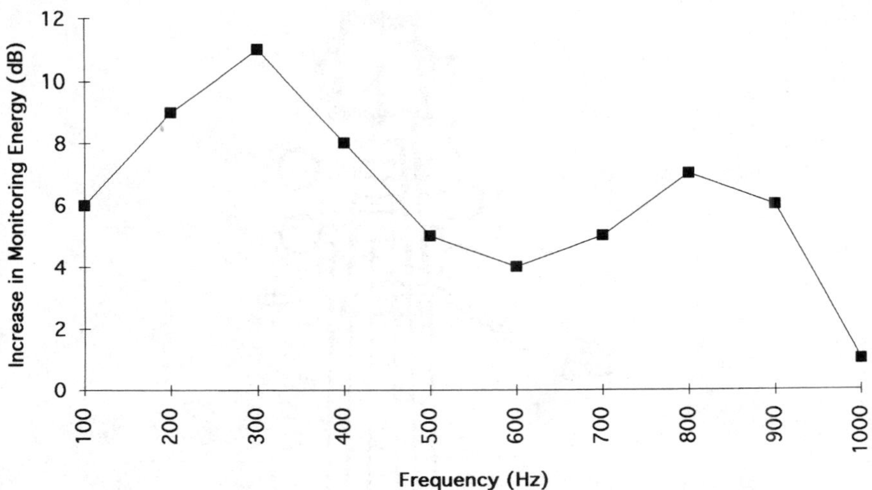

Figure 8–4. Low-frequency improvement when the acoustic monitoring device (shown in Figure 8–3) is used.

Table 8–1. Effect of Risers on Trumpet Intensity[a]

Frequency	Floor—Riser Difference
250	0
500	1
1000	3
2000	6
3000	5
4000	7
6000	6

[a]Measured at the level of the cellist.

is shown between the trumpet player placed on a riser as compared to being on the same level. There is a 5–7 dB high-frequency decrease in sound energy when placed on risers.

In addition to the protection of the musicians downwind, the overall level of trumpet players, when measured on the playing plane, are 2–4 dBA less intense when on risers. Anecdotally, trumpet players report that they tend to be less stressed when they play while on risers.

Various types of practice mutes are available for brass instruments and these have the general effect of reducing the overall sound levels. Depending on the model used, mutes can be quite frequency-specific, and musicians tend to try several models before they find one that is optimal for their style of playing. Because the more intense sounds of brass instruments are directional (away from the musician), practice mutes are more for the neighbors than for the brass players themselves. Electronic mutes can also be used that not only function as an acoustic attenuator, but also can allow the musician to monitor the music electronically through headphones. The listening level, simulated playing environment, and even degree of reverberation can be individually selected.

Finally, an innovation that has been of great use for French horn players is the use of a reflective baffle to their rear that is angled back at 45° to the floor. This baffle serves to reflect the higher frequency components of their music to the audience and, incidentally, is a welcome protector for the trumpet players who are unfortunately placed to their rear.

Woodwinds

The woodwind category is made up of clarinets, flutes, oboes, and bassoons, as the major representatives. These instruments can be played in in a wide range of venues, such as in large orchestras or with small jazz and blues bands. In orchestral environments, woodwinds are typically near the front of the orchestra but situated in front of the brass or percussion sections. In jazz and blues environments, they can be in front of speakers or near the drummer.

The ER-15 earplug is recommended for jazz and blues performing venues, and vented/tuned earplugs for the orchestral environments.

The rationale for the use of the vented/tuned earplugs in an orchestra is similar to that for the large stringed instruments—namely, to attenuate the high-frequency music energy from other instruments to the rear. The broader band ER-15 earplugs are more appropriate for the more varied music sources in a jazz or blues band.

The only alteration in an orchestral environment for woodwind players that is typically not used is the seating in a location that is completely unobstructed from the audience. With woodwind instruments, the sound emanates from the first noncovered finger hole, and as such may be "lost" between the legs and music stands of other musicians. Placing woodwind players in an unobstructed location will allow a direct path for their sound. If the woodwinds' sound is obstructed, overplaying can and does result with the potential of a career-ending injury to the obicularis oris muscle that controls the embouchure. This is also a frequently stated concern of brass musicians.

In the jazz and blues environment, a woodwind player may be situated near a speaker or near the cymbals of the drum kit. In most jazz or blues bands, the drummer hits harder on the ride cymbal (on the dominant side—typically the right side) and the woodwind player should situate himself or herself away from that potential source of music exposure. It is usually the best strategy to situate oneself parallel to a speaker rather than to the front or to the rear of the speaker, as the enclosure wall affords some protection.

Percussion Instruments

Whereas there may be some flexibility in the specification of ear protection for other instrument categories, there is very little choice for most percussionists. The ER-25 earplug is the optimal ear protection. As will be discussed later in this chapter, too much ear protection may be as hazardous as too little. Excessive ear protection may result in wrist or arm damage, and too little may result in a progressive music-induced hearing loss.

For the full drum kit (with drums and cymbals), hitting the high hat cymbal with a drum stick can be the greatest potential threat to hearing. It is commonplace to find that the hearing in the left ear is worse for a right handed drummer because of the close proximity to the high hat (and the converse for left handed drummers). The high hat is the main cymbal for rock and roll, with the ride cymbal (on the dominant or, typically, right side) for jazz and blues. The high hat, as the name suggests, is about the diameter of a brimmed hat with two opposing cymbals facing each other. A pedal can be used to move them together or leave them apart. Rock and roll musicians tend to play with the high hats slightly apart, whereas blues and jazz musicians tend to have them apart only about 50% of the time. Figure 8–5 shows two spectra with the high

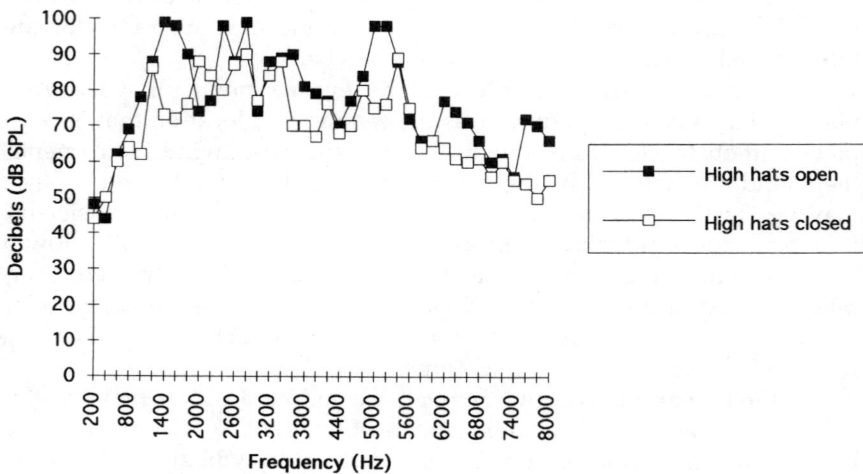

Figure 8–5. Two spectra of hitting the same high hat cymbal—open versus closed.

hats closed and with the high hats open. Note the increased spectral bandwidth and increased intensity when the high hats are left open. Although not shown in these spectra, the duration of the sound of the open high hat will be longer.

The positioning of the high hats is a matter of taste (and music style), and little can be done to convince a drummer to change his or her taste other than by education. However, many drummers are willing to play with a closed position high hat during practice sessions or even to use a muffling practice pad in between the two opposing faces of the high hat cymbal.

Another innovation that derives from the military, has recently been resurrected for drummers (and electric bass players) called a shaker (Futuresonics—see Appendix II). Shakers were originally designed to assess the hull integrity of submarines by mechanical vibrations. As shown in Figure 8–6, these devices look like large hockey pucks and can be bolted to the underside of a seat or the floor (or more commonly bolted to a piece of plywood that is placed on the floor). During playing, low-frequency vibrational feedback is available to the musician, providing him or her with better monitoring. Drummers using this device, tend not to play as loud with a subsequent reduction in the level of the music, and this potentially decreases risk of arm and wrist injury.

Drummers, doing studio work, frequently are required to use a *click track* in order to set the rate and maintain the rhythm of the music. A click track is typically provided by use of headphones; however, this approach degrades the monitoring of the higher frequency components of the music. A useful alternative is to transduce the click track through a pair of broadband (body aid style hearing aid) receivers. A common set-up is

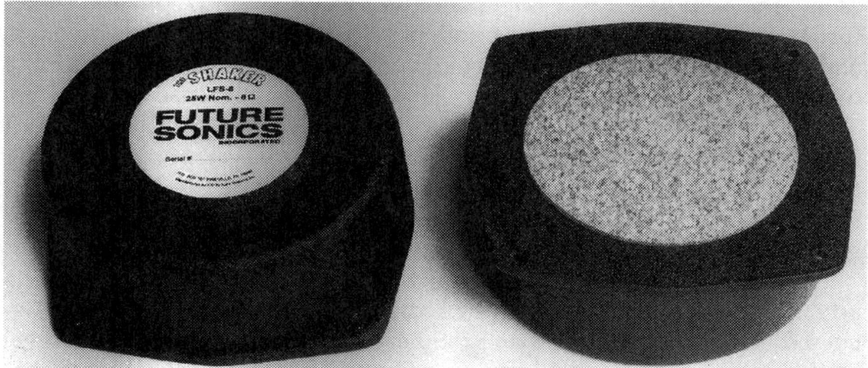

Figure 8–6. Shakers enhance the low-frequency vibrational feedback thus improving the monitoring for drummers and bass players. (Photograph courtesy of Futuresonics.)

to couple a pair of N-response (220 ohm) receivers to a Y-cord and receive the click tract from the monitor or click track source. The advantage of having a binaural fitting of the click track is that the intensity level can be set lower, while maintaining the same perception of loudness.

Finally, drummers can use the effect of their stapedial reflex to their advantage. If a loud sound is about to occur, such as by hitting a cymbal, the drummer can begin humming just prior to and through the length of the impulse. Such humming serves to elicit the stapedial reflex, thus providing some additional temporary ear protection. A discussion of the properties of the stapedial reflex can be found in Chapter 1.

Amplified Instruments

Musicians in amplified environments usually have a more flexible work environment than those who work in an orchestra. Rock, blues, and jazz musicians tend to work for themselves and are considered self-employed. Unlike many orchestral musicians, they may have some control over the instrument set-up. Therefore, recommendations of an environmental change for reducing the potential for music exposure are more frequently followed. There will be a discussion of some of the characteristics of self-employed musicians in Chapter 9.

These musicians should be situated either away from loud speakers or parallel to the enclosures as this will afford some protection. In those cases where loud speakers are oriented toward the musicians in order to obtain "side-wash," the speakers should be elevated. The intensity chosen by sound engineers if speakers are elevated is lower than if the loud speakers are on the floor. Figure 8–7 shows this phenomenon where a 6–8 dB low-frequency loss of energy is created by optimal coupling with the floor.

Optimal floor coupling means that the low-frequency sound energy "sees" the floor as a lower impedence pathway than the room and therefore takes this route. This low-frequency energy is lost to the performers and the audience. Many sound engineers compensate by turning up the overall level by 6–8 dB to re-establish an appropriate sense of loudness. They would be able to accomplish this same goal, with less overall intensity, if they merely equalize the amplification system by enhancing the low-frequency intensity level while maintaining the mid- and high-frequency levels. Elevating the loud speakers would obviate the need for such equalization.

The act of elevating loud speakers can also be to the performer's advantage by making use of their directional characteristics (as discussed in Chapter 3). Increasing the height of loud speakers to the level of the performer's ear will improve the monitoring of the higher frequency components that can be quite directional. Such an alteration can allow the sound engineer to decrease the overall sound level emanating from the loud speaker.

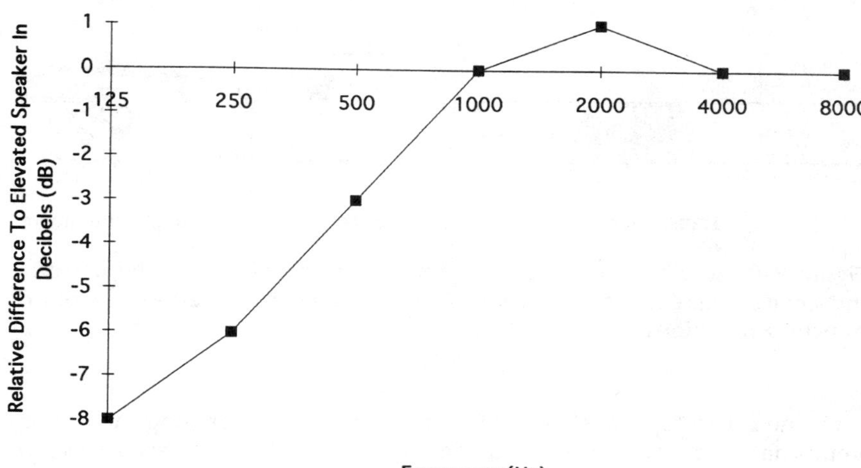

Figure 8–7. Low-frequency loss of sound energy from the room due to the loudspeaker enclosure being in contact with the floor. (From "Four Environmental Techniques to Reduce the Effect of Music Exposure on Hearing," by M. Chasin & J. Chong, 1995, *Medical Problems of Performing Artists, 10,* p. 67. Copyright 1995 by Hanley & Belfus, Inc. Reprinted with permission.)

In a large performance hall, loud speakers can be moved from the stage to a position in the hall. Because of the precedence effect discussed in Chapter 7, a 50 msec delay must be used with the loud speakers located in the hall so that the listeners will perceive the music to be emanating from the stage and not the loud speakers. Commercially available devices are available for such an application.

Shakers, such as that shown in Figure 8–6, can also be useful for electric bass players to provide better monitoring of their music as well as that of the drummer.

As an alternative to the ER-15 earplugs appropriate for most musicians who play amplified music, earphones that replace stage monitors are also an option. These earphones are custom or noncustom in-the-ear hearing aid shells that use a broadband receiver that can handle high-levels with minimal distortion. These are coupled via a wire to an FM receiver worn on the belt or under the clothes. The necessary music is mixed by the sound engineer and transmitted back to the musician so that there will be optimal monitoring. The musician is free to move about the stage because of the wireless nature of the transmission. Figure 8–8 shows a schematic of a custom earphone system.

Because the effects of the environment are minimized when these earphones are used, the sound levels at the ear are significantly lower than if the musicians were using conventional sound field monitoring systems. Figure 8–9 depicts two monitoring scenarios during a live per-

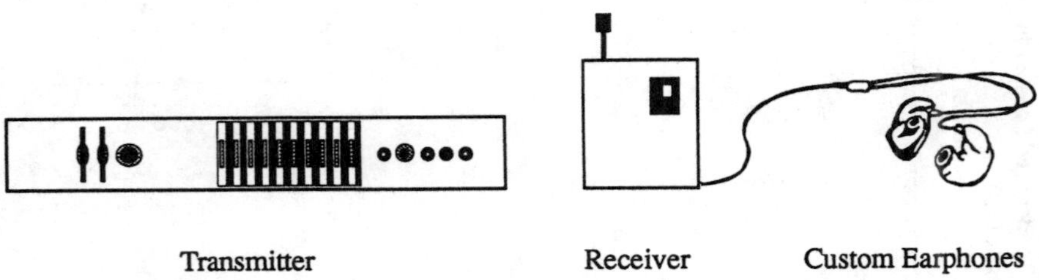

Figure 8–8. Schematic of earphones that allow the effects of the performing environment to be minimized. They are available in either custom or noncustom versions.

formance. The top panel denotes high sound levels on stage with conventional stage monitors, while the lower panel illustrates a reduced sound level when custom earphones are used.

Several manufacturers market such a system, and while they can be costly, custom earphones are gaining popularity. A list of some suppliers of these devices is found in Appendix II.

A less costly "hard wired" system can be used by coupling a pair of broad band hearing aid receivers (such as an N-response, 220 ohm) to standard (body aid style) earmolds and connecting this to an equalizer/amplifier that can be adjusted for overall gain and frequency response shaping. This in turn can be connected to a pressure zone microphone (PZM) placed in the center of the stage. Such a system has been successfully utilized, especially for drummers with an existing music-related hearing loss.

Vocalists

Classically trained sopranos can generate levels in excesss of 115 dB SPL. It is doubtful if any other register of vocalist can consistently generate such high levels. A typical question in a case history should therefore be a query if they are classically trained soprano singers.

By far, the primary concern of vocalists is related to vocal strain. Blues and jazz singers frequently complain of sore throats after long sets, especially in smoky environments. While part of the problem is the air quality, their situation can be ameliorated by the use of an earplug that creates a slight occlusion effect.

Vocalists are divided into two categories: solo and nonsolo. Solo vocalists can be found in classical environments and may be accompanied by relatively quiet instruments. The vented/tuned earplug is the most appropriate protection in this case. As will be discussed in the next section, such an earplug is more for improved monitoring than reduction of the music level.

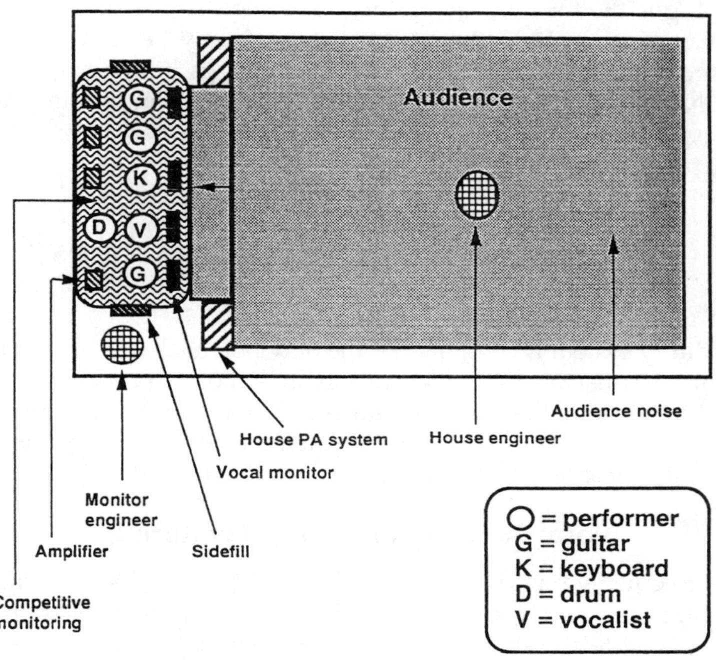

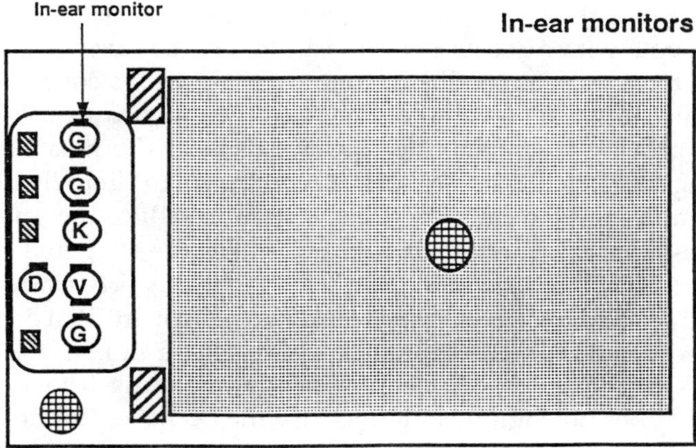

Figure 8–9. Two monitoring scenarios: one with traditional stage monitoring (top) and the other with custom earphones (bottom). (From "Protecting The Professional Ear: Conservation Strategies And Devices," by J. W. Hall & M. Santucci, 1995, *Hearing Journal, 48*, p. 44. Copyright 1995 by Williams & Wilkins. Reprinted with permission.)

Nonsolo vocalists, typically found in pop bands, are susceptible to the same sources of music exposure than their instrumental colleagues. Because of the wide range of music sources on stage, the wide band ER-15 earplug is the form of ear protection of choice. As in the case of the solo performer, a slight degree of occlusion may be useful, and it is therefore recommended that the ER-15 earplugs be made with short canals. Nonsolo vocalists will also gain an improved monitoring (as well as some protection from the various sources of music) by using the custom earphones as shown in Figure 8–8.

TWO HEARING/NONHEARING INTERACTIONS

(or "My Wrist Sings the Blues")

The auditory system is certainly not the only potential area of damage for musicians. Entire clinics have been set up, based on a sports injury model, to provide rehabilitation services and prevention education to musicians. Two forms of musician injury can be related directly to improper auditory monitoring. These are vocal strain–nodules and wrist–arm injury.

Vocal Strain and Hearing Monitoring

Singers frequently report vocal strain, especially after a long set or if they are required to sing in a smoky environment. Although vocal strain is primarily related to the singing intensity and length of singing time, vocal strain may also be related to monitoring. Monitoring of one's own voice is necessary for the proper speaking and singing intensity. It is well known that people with a sensorineural hearing loss, because of a lack of monitoring, tend to speak loudly. In contrast, those with a conductive loss tend to speak at a quieter level since they hear their own voice as louder.

Improving the monitoring of a singer's voice during a performance by creating a slight occlusion effect has been shown to clinically decrease vocal strain, and in a few cases, has been shown to reduce the severity of vocal nodules. This is a very exciting area of current research and investigations are underway that seek to assess a wide range of voice-related measures as a result of improved monitoring caused by a slight artificial occlusion.

The vented/tuned earplug has been of use in many jazz and blues venues to reduce vocal strain. Strictly speaking, the vented/tuned earplug does not significantly increase the occlusion effect. This earplug has a vent-associated resonance (see Chapter 5) that creates a mild low-frequency amplification. And it is this slight amplification that serves to improve the singers' monitoring of their own voice. The ER-15 earplug has also been modified to create a slight occlusion effect by intentionally shortening the length of the bore. The shortened ER-15 earplug is more appropriate for rock and roll singers.

Wrist–Arm Injury and Hearing Monitoring

Drummers tend to be aware of the potential of music-related hearing loss. It is commonplace for them to have read in the popular press that drummers require hearing protection, and the most available type is the industrial strength earplugs. Wrist and/or arm strain is the number one reason for drummers seeking medical help. These two occurrences can be related.

The following scenario is commonly found with drummers: A drummer starts to wear industrial-strength ear protection such as foam plugs, and after about 6 months, arm and/or wrist pain begins.

This problem can be directly related to the wrong ear protection. Industrial-strength foam earplugs attenuate the higher frequency energy to such an extent that there may be a loss of monitoring of the energy from the cymbals and snare drum. Table 8–2 shows the intensity of a drummer hitting a practice drum pad with no ear protection, with the wrong ear protection (foam earplugs), and with the ER-25 earplugs.

Note that the hitting intensity of the "no ear protection" and the "ER-25 earplug" conditions are similar, whereas that of the "industrial foam earplug" is much greater. In this case, the loss of high-frequency monitoring caused by the foam earplugs caused the drummer to hit the practice pad harder, increasing the potential for arm and/or wrist injury.

SUMMARY

Table 8–3 summarizes many of the strategies and devices that can be used to minimize the potential for hearing loss from music sources. The relevant figures referred to in Table 8–3 are useful for the counseling of the musician. Laminated copies of those figures are used routinely in explaining the characteristics of music, strategies, and devices to the musician.

Table 8–2. Intensity of Hitting Drum Pad with Poor, Good, and No Ear Protection

Ear Protection	dBA
Industrial foam earplug	113
ER-25 earplug	104
No ear protection	103

Table 8–3 Strategies and Devices for Reducing Hearing Loss in Musicians

Instrument	Problems	Solutions	Figures
Small strings	Overhang	Move away from overhang	8–2
	Own music	ER-15 earplugs	5–4, 5–5
	Practicing	Practice mute	
Large strings	Brass section	Vented/tuned earplugs	5–4, 5–5
		Brass on risers	4–9
	Monitoring	Acoustic monitor tube (cello)	8–4
Brass	Other musician complaints	Brass on riser	Table 8–1
	Practice	Acoustic/electronic practice mutes	
	Other brass	Baffles	
Woodwinds	Instruments to rear	Brass on risers	4–9
		Earplugs	5–4, 5–5
	Amplified Instruments	Move parallel to speakers	
Percussion	High hats	Practice pads	
		Closed high hats	8–5
	Monitoring	Shakers	8–6
		Custom earphones	8–8
	Wrist strain	ER-25	Table 8–2
Amplified Instruments	Speakers	Move parallel to speakers	
		Elevate speakers	8–7
		ER-15 earplugs	5–4, 5–5
	Monitoring	Shakers	8–6
		Custom earphones	8–8
Vocalists	Speakers	ER-15 or vented/ tuned earplugs	5–4, 5–5
	Monitoring	Custom earphones	8–8

CHAPTER 9

The Human Performance Approach to Prevention

INTRODUCTION

An important aspect of the treatment of musicians and the prevention of hearing loss is the work environment and the associated management/performing artist dynamics. As will be discussed in this chapter, musicians have a large stake in their physical well being (including the prevention of hearing loss) and this desire for optimal health is occasionally at odds with the work environment they may find themselves in.

THE HUMAN PERFORMANCE MODEL

Unlike most occupational health problems, the issue of prevention of hearing loss among musicians serves as an example whereby the indi-

---

John Chong—an accomplished concert pianist—wrote this chapter. It serves as an epilogue as well as a "musician manifesto." Dr. Chong is the medical director and founder of Canada's first performing arts medicine program at the Centre for Human Performance and Health Promotion, in Hamilton, Ontario, known to most musicians as the "Musicians' Clinic."

vidual's dependence on hearing throughout his or her occupational career is a paramount principle of prevention. As discussed in the previous chapters, the exposure levels among various types of music exposure from individual performances to large scale rock productions often exceed the exposure limits defined by various regulatory bodies across the world (see, for example, Embleton, 1995).

The natural history of sound exposure in a musician's career begins usually at an early age often paralleling that of the development of speech and language skills. Enhancement of musical performance skills often accelerates to peak performance in early childhood and adolescence. This is in sharp contrast to the average industrial workers who take on a job in their twenties and excel very little after that time period.

This implies that the professional musician has a significant cumulative sound exposure before even entering the performing arts workplaces and may have already suffered significant hearing loss. The experience of the Musicians' Clinic in Canada only echoes this rather startling fact that nine out of ten musicians that present with work-related musculoskeletal disorders to a treatment facility also have measurable hearing loss (Chasin & Chong, 1992).

The traditional labor/management model of prevention does not necessarily apply to hearing loss among musicians, as the problem has developed prior to the professional musician's participation in a traditional labor management marketplace.

Therefore, the opportunities for prevention lie in understanding the development of the performing artist at an early age, and the likelihood of success of these interventions predates the venues that one would associate with professional employment.

As the performing artist develops from a student to semiprofessional and to professional levels, the nature of employment is usually of a self-employed status for economic reasons. This trend alters once again the nature of intervention opportunities. In a salaried, or more organized work environment, group intervention would be favored; however, where self-employed workers tend to be the rule, an individual-based approach would be more efficient.

Because of recent economic changes in the arts and entertainment industry, self-employed individuals working in small to medium-sized work groups tend to be the rule. Gone are the days of the large-scale salaried orchestra members as has been the tradition in Europe.

With the advent of electronic technology and the rapid dissemination of entertainment medium through video and compact discs, small self-employed groups with computerized electronic music systems have proliferated in the last ten years. This again focuses the potential for prevention to an individual-based model rather than a large-scale group intervention one.

Therefore, the impact of computerized and electronic technology in the arts and entertainment industry cannot be underestimated. The nature of the production and performing arts indeed has been changed in a profound and dramatic fashion.

Combining these various factors that are based on the nature of career development, the natural history of the target health condition, and the socioeconomic changes in the arts and entertainment industry, one can see quite clearly that a prevention model based on individual human performance is better suited than a traditional labor/management approach.

The fact that the performing artist is unable to function without an excellent sense of hearing acuity is indeed an advantage to the hearing health care professional interested in preventing this type of health problem. The musician literally cannot function to an optimal degree and pursue gainful employment without the best possible hearing as well as physical function throughout his or her entire career. The implications of the aging process among this population are extremely important, as the career of musicians not only begins very early but extends to the end of their lives.

Therefore examples of successful preventative interventions lie in a clinic-based model whereby individual musicians who choose a comprehensive health evaluation for musculoskeletal problems, performance anxiety, and hearing assessment are amenable to a multidisciplinary prevention approach. In our clinical experience many vocalists and instrumentalists are keenly aware and interested enough in their hearing abilities to implement stategies to prevent further decline of their hearing status. Practical approaches to exposure reduction at the source and at the musician's ear have been covered in Chapters 5, 7, and 8. These strategies and devices are as equally important for students and young developing musicians as for the professional or semiprofessional musician.

Other attempts have been carried out based on a labor/management model in large-scale arts and entertainment venues and more often than not these have been unsuccessful for political and economic reasons. These large-scale productions have well-documented excessive sound exposure levels (see Chapter 2) and are quite profitable in terms of gross cash flow on a day-to-day basis. It has been our experience that these political and economic concerns far outweigh those of the health and safety of the instrumentalists and singers and therefore prevention efforts have essentially been ignored.

Nevertheless, the individual musicians and singers at risk have an option to seek clinical assistance at any time concerning their hearing health. Many of these individuals have sought help for audiological assessment and advice in terms of primary prevention. This model has proven successful in many situations (Chong et al., 1991).

There have been some exceptions, and a trend toward increased cooperation is being observed in some performance venues. Certainly a major step will be the development of performing arts guidelines such as those recently implemented in Ontario by the province's Ministry of Labour (1993). In some sense, the actual content of these guidelines is only of secondary importance. The primary benefit may be the process whereby representatives of management and performing artists negotiate for a safe and long-lasting working environment.

Vocalists and instrumentalists have found customized personal hearing protective devices described in Chapter 5 to be extremely useful not only for reducing sound exposure, but also for improving musical performance. In a studio or individual practice environment, the human peformance prevention model is indeed highly successful because of the degree of control offered to the musical performer.

ROLE OF GOVERNMENT AND REGULATORY AGENCIES

The issue in general of noise-induced hearing loss in industry has been a topic of much scientific and political debate. Traditional efforts have been directed toward hearing conservation programs and audiometric measurement rather than reducing exposures at the source. The cost effectiveness of this passive secondary prevention has been promoted by numerous authors (see, for example, Sataloff & Sataloff, 1995). The role of government and regulatory agencies has followed the secondary prevention model as often as the economic nonfeasibility of primary intervention has been used by employers to avoid reducing sound exposure levels at the source. Recent technological advances, however, make such exposure-reduction techniques more cost effective and potentially applicable in more workplaces. Unfortunately in the arts and entertainment industry, the nature of the exposure is not only the art form but also the hazard. This contradiction unfortunately leaves not only the performer but the audience in a dilemma.

Practical strategies to isolate musicians from excessive levels of sound exposure have been tried in orchestral and band situations to a limited degree. The use of risers and acoustical separation are of some benefit in limited situations. In the recording studio environment this approach is quite useful; however, on a large theater stage or orchestral stage, these approaches have been met with less approval from management and even some musicians. The problem with acoustic isolation and the lack of feeling of the performance emsemble is problematic with some types of acoustic strategies. However, the appropriate customized hearing protective devices are usable in a wide range of music exposures.

It is important to stress that the exposure of the individual musician can vary from the practice studio to the teaching studio, to concert hall stage to recording studio, and repeated again in a number of cycles through a working day. Therefore, the individual hearing protective devices approach is far more acceptable than other strategies, in our clinical experience.

Government and regulatory agencies have often recommended the traditional industrial type of earplugs at an action level of usually 85–90 dBA in most jurisdictions. The enforcement of such recommendations is generally lax, however. The hearing protective device that is worn more often than not offers less protection than the device that theoretically provides maximum attenuation with problems of discomfort and isolation (Alberti, 1982).

It has been the practice of government and regulatory agencies to legislate the "internal responsibility system" that essentially leaves the onus on individual workers to protect themselves. This assumes that each and every individual worker has a fundamental understanding of the risk of overexposure to excessive acoustical energy and the natural history of noise-induced hearing loss.

NEED FOR EDUCATION OF MUSICIANS

Recently, sensitization to the profound risks and tragedy of hearing loss in highly talented performers has brought about organizations such as HEAR (Hearing Education and Awareness for Rockers) in the United States and FHARTS (Foundation for Health in the Arts) in Canada (see Appendix II). These are nonprofit organizations with the mission of sensitizing performing artists to the issue of hearing loss and other arts-related hazards.

These organizations are early in their development and key individuals have brought forward their own personal histories to highlight the seriousness of the health concerns. Musicians such as Pete Townsend (of The Who) have made no secret of their individual problems with hearing loss and tinnitus. They have literally and singlehandedly promoted their own health impairment selflessly to bring attention to the issue. These organizations are crucial in the educational network by disseminating information to smaller arts organizations such as orchestras and small instrumental groups.

The role of instrument manufacturers and the electronic arts and entertainment industry has yet to join this educational effort to a large degree. Manufacturers of musical instruments and those working in the development of the technology surrounding music must begin to collaborate and fund these educational efforts. This is not unlike the tobacco industry funding antismoking campaigns, and large-scale economic participation has yet to be realized.

THE MUSICIAN AS ACOUSTIC ATHLETE

Based on the above key concepts, musicians in their artistic development would ideally need to be educated about the inherent risk of excessive sound exposure during their careers.

Educational efforts have been carried out in numerous educational institutions in the United States and Canada since the early 1980s and have been met with a large degree of acceptance. Examples of this include conservatories and faculties of music. Smaller groups including elementary music programs have been most interested. This latter group includes music teachers employed by school boards and private music schools. The opportunities for educating high school music students often have been in place because of the awareness of their teachers. The target population of musicians between the ages of 10 and 30 can be reached through this type of organized and cooperative effort with educational institutions. Priorities in this area need to be developed with adequate funding and resources from the relevant government agencies and performing arts industries.

There is now an increasing trend of accepting the human performance prevention model for a number of reasons. Although the immediate impact of interventions of devices such as custom earplugs cannot be immediately realized from a health perspective, the benefits to musical performance are, in contrast, readily perceived. This unique opportunity can be seized upon by the clinician to capture the performing artists' attention at this vulnerable age. Also, the fact that performers of wide acclaim have adopted a healthy behavior toward the prevention of hearing loss before the development of serious impairment sets an excellent example to the younger musician before it is too late. Many influential musicians that have demonstrated a health promotion behavior early in their careers have expressed the benefits of not only health accrual but economic spin-offs to this approach.

Therefore, there is a rapidly developing trend in the arts community to one of health-seeking behaviors based on an awareness of the seriousness of the problem discussed in this text. The importance of accurate and timely education about the long-term health implications of hearing loss and the practical simplicity of prevention cannote be overstated. The past has been clouded with denial and secrecy concerning this issue. Musicians have skirted the issue of hearing loss and espouse the attitude of occupational Darwinism—that is, survival of the fittest. This fatalistic attitude of accepting inherent risks of their occupation has led many prominent performing artists to significant disability and career termination. Simply put, the musician with a significant hearing loss is unable to perform at the professional levels required to be competitive and drops out of the work force. This key fact allows the clinician to intervene not from a theoretical model but from a practical problem-solving approach.

EDUCATION OF HEALTH PROFESSIONALS

The education of physicians, nurses, and therapists has been extremely weak in the discipline of occupational health and prevention. The economics of health care have favored an illness treatment system of health delivery rather than a health promotion perspective. This only adds further pressure on health professionals to become aware and educate themselves on how to intervene in a timely and cost-effective manner. The development of arts medicine clinics across North America and Europe offers this opportunity for health professionals to practice this craft and hopefully stem the tide of this widespread occupational health problem in the arts and entertainment community.

However, the opportunity for medical students interested in this unique area of practice is indeed limited at this point and organizations such as the Performing Arts Medicine Association and the International Arts Medicine Association have initiated efforts to provide opportunities for educating health professionals on such issues.

The discipline of arts medicine is in its infancy and the problem of hearing loss among musicians is a priority health problem. Practical strategies of intervening with a human performance prevention model offer the arts medicine clinician an important role in identifying and preventing this health problem. The beneficiaries of these efforts—the young developing musicians—need to be reached in a systematic and organized fashion by music educators.

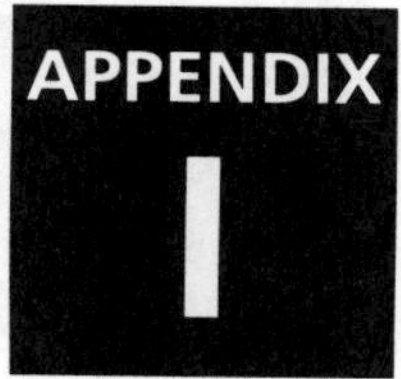

Clinical Information

This appendix contains information that can be used in the clinical assessment of those in the performing arts. Several tables and figures are reproduced here for convenience.

CONVERSION CHART

A musical note-to-frequency conversion table for the tempered musical scale is provided and can be used to directly translate REM resonant date to equivalent musical notes.

FIGURE REPRODUCTION

The following figures are reproduced for convenience of reference: The optimal hearing protection chart from Chapter 5; the attenuation characteristics of four hearing protectors from Chapter 5; and the summary sheet of relevant solutions and figures from Chapter 8.

SAMPLE REPORT

A sample report for a clinical assessment of a musician is also provided. The figures referred to in the sample report are Figures 3–5, 3–9, and 4–4.

C_0	16		C_3	131		C_6	1047	
		17			139			1109
D_0	18		D_3	147		D_6	1175	
		19			156			1245
E_0	21		E_3	165		E_6	1319	
F_0	22		F_3	175		F_6	1397	
		23			185			1480
G_0	25		G_3	196		G_6	1568	
		26			208			1661
A_0	28		A_3	220		A_6	1760	
		29			233			1865
B_0	31		B_3	247		B_6	1976	
C_1	33		C_4	262		C_7	2093	
		35			277			2218
D_1	37		D_4	294		D_7	2349	
		39			311			2489
E_1	41		E_4	330		E_7	2637	
F_1	44		F_4	349		F_7	2794	
		46			370			2960
G_1	49		G_4	392		G_7	3136	
		52			415			3322
A_1	55		A_4	440		A_7	3520	
		58			466			3729
B_1	62		B_4	494		B_7	3951	
C_2	65		C_5	523		C_8	4186	
		69			554			4435
D_2	73		D_5	587		D_8	4699	
		78			622			4978
E_2	82		E_5	659		E_8	5274	
F_2	87		F_5	698		F_8	5588	
		92			740			5920
G_2	98		G_5	784		G_8	6272	
		104			831			6645
A_2	110		A_5	880		A_8	7040	
		117			932			7459
B_2	123		B_5	988		B_8	7902	

Figure I–1. Conversion chart of musical notes-to-frequency. Notes on the piano span from A_0 to C_8, with sharps/flats being offset. (From *The Acoustical Foundations of Music* [p. 153] by J. Backus, 1977, New York: W. W. Norton & Company, Inc. Copyright 1977 by W. W. Norton & Company, Inc. Adapted with permission.)

Table I–1. Optimal Hearing Protection for Musicians

Instrument	Auditory Damage	Earplugs
Reeded woodwinds	Brass section to rear	ER-15 Vented/tuned
Flutes	Flutes (>105 dB SPL)	ER-15 Vented/tuned
Small strings	Small strings (>110 dB SPL)	ER-15
Large strings	Brass section to rear	Vented/tuned
Brass	Brass	Vented/tuned
Percussion	Percussion (high hats)	ER-25
Vocalists Solo	Soprano (>115 dB SPL)	Vented/tuned
Nonsolo	Other instruments	ER-15
Amplified Instruments	Speakers/monitors	ER-15

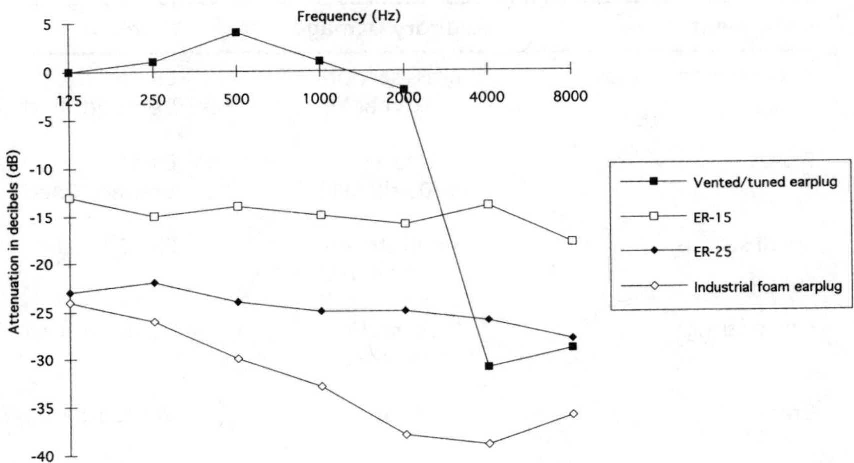

Figure I–2. Attenuation characteristics of the ER-15, ER-25, and the vented/tuned earplugs. The industrial earplug data is also given for comparison purposes. (From "A Clinically Efficient Hearing Protection Program for Musicians," by M. Chasin & J. Chong, 1992, *Medical Problems of Performing Artists, 7,* p. 41. Copyright 1992 by Hanley & Belfus, Inc. Adapted with permission.)

Table I–2. Strategies and Devices for Reducing Hearing Loss in Musicians

Instrument	Problems	Solutions	Figures
Small strings	Overhang	Move away from overhang	8–2
	Own music	ER-15 earplugs	5–4, 5–5
	Practicing	Practice mute	
Large strings	Brass section	Vented/tuned earplugs	5–4, 5–5
		Brass on risers	4–9
	Monitoring	Acoustic monitor tube (cello)	8–4
Brass	Other musician complaints	Brass on riser	Table 8–1
	Practice	Acoustic/electronic practice mutes	
	Other brass	Baffles	
Woodwinds	Instruments to rear	Brass on risers	4–9
		Earplugs	5–4, 5–5
	Amplified Instruments	Move parallel to speakers	
Percussion	High hats	Practice pads	
		Closed high hats	8–5
	Monitoring	Shakers	8–6
		Custom earphones	8–8
	Wrist strain	ER-25	Table 8–2
Amplified Instruments	Speakers	Move parallel to speakers	
		Elevate speakers	8–7
		ER-15 earplugs	5–4, 5–5
	Monitoring	Shakers	8–6
		Custom earphones	8–8
Vocalists	Speakers	ER-15 or vented/ tuned earplugs	5–4, 5–5
	Monitoring	Custom earphones	8–8

re: Michael X
(instruments: flute, clarinet, and saxophone)

Audiometry

Audiometry indicated a very mild high-frequency notch at 6000 Hz (4–5 white notes above the highest note on the piano keyboard), which is consistent with early music exposure. This loss has more to do with the anatomy of the inner ear rather than with the music spectra; however, the various music spectra can be a secondary factor.

It should be pointed out that this very mild notch at 6000 Hz can be thought of as a result of the way we test hearing. The softest sounds that can be heard across a range of frequencies (which is the audiogram) can be thought of as an *equal loudness contour*. These equal loudness contours tend to "flatten out" as the presentation level increases—such that if measured at a typical playing or speaking intensity, the audiogram would be completely normal. The very mild notch should therefore be thought of as only an early warning sign of potential future hearing loss and not as current problem.

Musical Environment

It was reported that among the various venues, auditory damage may also originate from the trumpet section to the rear and from occasional picollo and flute to the left ear. It is recommended that whenever possible, the flute and picollo be on his right side (blowing away from Michael) or if this is not possible, angled away from Michael's left ear. The trumpets should be on risers, as the higher frequency harmonic energy of the trumpet can be very intense and, because of the bell, this damaging high-frequency energy is highly directional. That is, if the output of the trumpet is measured at a point 30° below the playing plane of the trumpet, the intensity of the higher frequency energy can be 6 decibels (dB) less than at the playing plane of the trumpet. If risers are used for the trumpet, much of the damaging high frequency energy will literally go over Michael's head.

Spectral Analysis

Flute

A low F (with a fundamental frequency of 349 Hz) was played at a mezzo forte level and the fundamental had an intensity of 88 dB SPL (Sound Pressure Level) as measured in the right ear canal. The higher frequency harmonic energy of this note was less intense (i.e., the first harmonic was only 73 dB SPL at about 700 Hz).

It is interesting to note that the flute is acting as a one-half wavelength resonator with harmonics being integer multiples of the fundamental frequency. When the same note F_4 (349 Hz) was played at a forte level, the level rose only 4 dB to 94 dB SPL. It is also interesting that the first harmonic of this note was also approximately 94 dB SPL. This relative high-frequency boost when playing very loudly is more characteristic of reeded woodwinds but the flute also has this characteristic to a lesser degree—specfically the first harmonic at 700 Hz [F_5 (698 Hz)] rose 21 dB from mezzo forte to forte, whereas the fundamental only rose 4 dB. This indicates that, even in the flute, there is a high-frequency spectral cue that is indicative of the playing loudness. In this case, taking off this high-frequency cue (such as with a recommendation of an industrial strength plug) may cause Michael to lose his loudness monitoring ability.

This is only a hypothesis, however. Although this cue is definitely here (and caused by harmonic distortion or combinatorial aggregate), Michael may not be using it. I would suspect that with someone as experienced as Michael, he may rely more on subglottal pressure and embouchure (obicularis oris tension) rather than on audition of the higher frequency information.

A higher frequency note was also assessed that is more in the playing range of the flute. This was A_5 (880 Hz). When played mezzo forte, a level of 100 dB SPL was found for the fundamental energy, with a rapid fall off of the higher frequency harmonic energy (at about 1800 Hz). When played forte, a level of 108 dB SPL was found for the fundamental with a modest fall off for the higher frequency harmonic structure. There is a relative increase of harmonic energy in the forte condition but only a 16 dB increase. Clearly for this note [A_5 (880 Hz)], prolonged exposure can damage hearing.

Comparing a lower frequency note [F_5 (698 Hz)] with the higher frequency note [A_5 (880 Hz)], the relative harmonic energy increase, (due to an increase in playing intensity), of the lower note was 17 dB (= 21 dB − 4 dB) and that of the higher note was 8 dB (= 16 dB − 8 dB). The high-frequency intensity cue is still apparent but I am doubtful if Michael utilizes it.

B flat clarinet

The clarinet (3.5 strength reed) was assessed in the same fashion as that of the flute: mezzo forte vs. forte with both a lower register note and a higher register note. The lower register note [G_3 (196 Hz)] was measured at 70 dB SPL for the fundamental and 68 dB SPL for the first harmonic (just below 600 Hz). This indicates that the clarinet is functioning as a quarter wavelength resonator with odd number multiples of the fundamental being the harmonics. When played at a forte level there was no measureable change in the fundamental (70 dB SPL) but the first harmonic rose to 80 dB SPL—a 12 dB high-frequency relative increase when played at a more intense level. Neither level is potentially damaging, however. The degree of relative increase is caused by the distortion products of the vibrating reed, with the higher strength reeds having a greater level of distortion (i.e., greater reed strength results in a more nonlinear system).

The high-frequency note assessed was two octaves higher at [G_5 (784 Hz)]. Played at mezzo forte, the level was 77 dB SPL, with the first harmonic at 80 dB SPL. When played forte, a level of 102 dB SPL was obtained for both the fundamental and the first harmonic. The relative high-frequency increase for this note was negligible (3 dB for mezzo forte and 0 dB for forte). It seems that this phenomenon decreases as playing frequency increases. Even if Michael does utilize the high-frequency harmonic intensity cue to monitor his playing loudness, this utilization would have to fall off as playing frequency increases.

B flat Saxophone

A low register G_3 (196 Hz) was played mezzo forte and a level of 80 dB SPL was found, with the first higher harmonic being at about 392 Hz and 92 dB SPL. When played at a forte level, the fundamental only increased to 81 dB SPL, with the first resonance at about 392 Hz and being 95 dB SPL. The relative high frequency energy increase was only 2 dB.

When playing the next higher octave, G_4 (392 Hz) was played at a mezzo forte level, the fundamental was 95 dB SPL, and the first harmonic was also 95 dB SPL. When played forte, the level was 104 dB SPL and the first harmonic was 99 dB SPL. There was actually a 5 dB decrease in relative level when played at a more intense level.

Hearing Protection

The hearing protection of choice is the ER-15 earplug that uniformly attenuates all sound energy equally. In some of the quieter venues the ER-element may be removed from the earplug, which will result in the creation of a vented/tuned earplug (with a 3 mm inner diameter vent). In the vented/tuned condition all sound energy is passed unaffected; however, there is a 30 dB decrease in sound energy above 2000 Hz (one octave below the highest note on the piano keyboard). Michael will have to experiment with these earplugs to see which is best. The vented/tuned earplug may be useful if he is around high-frequency emphasis instruments such as trumpets, picollos, and cymbal percussion, as these earplugs will provide more protection for these higher frequency sounds (up to 30 dB) over the ER-15 (only 15 dB protection). However, if Michael feels that he is losing his loudness monitoring ability, he shold use the ER-15 earplugs.

Speaker/Monitor Change

When using a monitor or a speaker, both should be elevated from the floor. If on the floor, the low frequencies (that couple well with floor boards) will be absorbed by the floor and thereby be lost to the audience or monitoring. The sound engineer in trying to compensate will enhance the overall level because of the loss of loudness (loudness is a low-frequency perception phenomenon) with the result of a greater potential for hearing damage.

Michael expressed an interest in having his sound monitored as "full." This comment translates into a mid frequency enhancement on the equalizer board by 4–5 dB. It is suggested that on his own monitor channel that the higher frequencies also be enhanced, which will provide him with improved loudness perception for some of his instruments. This should be enhanced also by 6–8 dB. It should be pointed out that the high-frequency monitor channel should not be enhanced unless the mid-range frequencies also are enhanced. Without an enhancement in the 1000–2000 Hz region (corresponding to a feeling of greater "fullness" in the music), the high-frequency monitor boost will sound tinny and unnatural. He therefore will not need to play as intensely, thus reducing the overall potential for noise exposure. In addition, there will be less embouchure strain such that after a long set, he will be more relaxed and can enjoy his music more.

Sincerely,

Marshall Chasin, M.Sc., Reg. OSLA, Aud(C), FAAA
Audiologist

Resources and Service Development

This appendix contains resource addresses and a sample "proposal for service" that can be used in the development of a performing arts prevention program.

Custom (C) and Noncustom (NC) Earphones Manufacturers

Etymotic Research (NC)
61 Martin Lane
Elk Grove Village, IL 60007
USA

Future Sonics (C)
P.O. Box 187
1006 Holicong Road
Pineville, PA 18946-0187
USA

Sensaphonics Inc. (C)
660 North Milwaukee Avenue
Chicago, IL 60622
USA

Advocacy and Educational Organizations

Foundation for Health in the Arts
c/o Centre for Human Performance and Health Promotion
565 Sanatorium Road
Hamilton, Ontario, Canada, L9C 7N4

Hearing Education and Awareness for Rockers (HEAR)
P.O. Box 460847
San Francisco, CA 94146 USA

Better Hearing Institute (BHI)
P.O. Box 1840
Washington, DC 20013 USA

Canadian Hearing Society (CHS)
271 Spadina Road
Toronto, Ontario, Canada, M5R 2V3

Canadian Hearing Society (CHS)
271 Spadina Road
Toronto, Ontario, Canada, M5R 2V3

British Society of Audiology
80 Brighton Road
Reading, Berkshire RG6 1P5 UK

Sample Proposal to an Orchestra

This outline proposal has been used successfully and can be adapted for any local orchestras or bands.

XXX Hearing Health Care Proposal

Introduction to the Problem

Hearing loss from music exposure is identical to hearing loss from exposure to industrial noise. When it comes to hearing damage, the ear in all of its complexity cannot distinguish between noise and music. Both music and noise are merely vibrations in the air and, ultimately, neurological impulses in the auditory system.

Because of the similarity between noise exposure and music exposure, the Ontario Ministry of Labour recently formed a committee and in December, 1993, created guidelines that would protect the musician from long-term hearing loss caused by music. The Centre for Human Performance and Health Promotion (also referred to as the Musician's Clinic) served as professional consultants to the relevant subcommittee.

The following represents both the spirit and the available technology embodied in those guidelines. The proper application of the information contained in this proposal will ensure that musical quality is maintained while at the same time not sacrificing the integrity of the musician's hearing.

The Centre for Human Performance and Health Promotion has previously measured the intensity of many orchestras—both classical and modern—with startling results. For example, music levels on the right shoulder of the flute player in Canada's National Ballet have been measured at 126 dB (decibels), and in National Youth Orchestra rehearsals at 109 dB.

Research from industry has shown that prolonged exposure to sound levels over 85 dB can permanently damage your hearing. Clearly musicians are subject to levels of music that are far in excess of the level which their auditory systems can tolerate.

By its very nature hearing loss due to noise exposure is gradual and may take many years to notice. Even then, music exposure is noticed more as a loss of clarity rather than as one of loudness per se. Hearing loss from music (and noise) manifests itself in a characteristic pattern, with the greatest hearing loss around 4000 Hz; this corresponds to the top note on the piano keyboard. Gradually, the hearing loss progresses if music exposure is not reduced and becomes noted also in lower frequency regions—and eventually into the region of the fundamental energy of musical instruments. Initially, the higher frequency harmonics are only affected. Although this loss may not be crucial for a woodwind player (who relies on lower frequency "breathiness" cues in order to have a good tone), this would be disasterous for string musicians such as violin players. Violinists need to hear the higher frequency harmonic structure in order to play with a good quality of sound.

Some Solutions

Understandably, in order to prevent hearing loss, *education needs to be a cornerstone.* Such education is usually carried out within the confines of an audiometric assessment. Audiometric testing can be performed on site for the musicians—the results of which can be used to improve the monitoring of some musicians' playing. For example, the monitor on an electronically amplified instrument may not need to be as loud if it can be equalized, taking into account the musician's individual hearing ability.

A second aspect of any hearing loss prevention program is environmental manipulation. Other than the obvious example of the use of baffles for the isolation of certain impulse/percussive instruments, many subtle but effective position changes can be made.

To illustrate this point two examples follow. In the case of the overhang in the musicians' performance pit, acoustic damping may be advantageous for woodwinds but be disasterous for the strings. The damping material on the ceiling serves to attenuate the higher frequency energy. A violin section in this area would lose some of the higher frequency harmonic energy, which they so importantly require, whereas the clarinet section would have no problems in this position. Thus, moving the string section out of this area would be advantageous to their monitoring and playing ability.

A second example involves the trumpet section. Belled instruments are highly directional, but only for the higher frequency sounds. Elevating the tumpet section would have the effect of allowing all of the damaging higher frequency harmonic energy to literally go over the heads of the other musicians "downwind."

In addition to position changes, acoustic modifications can be made and/or altered in the performance pit.

A third aspect of a hearing protection program is the specification of personalized ear protection where required. The Centre for Human Performance and Health Promotion has developed techniques to assess ear protection requirements and has developed and modified ear protection that can be tuned precisely for the musician, taking individual factors into account such as playing style, reed strength, bow type, and performing positioning within the orchestra.

A range of hearing protection is available that has been designed specifically with the musician in mind. These include the ER-15, the ER-25, and the vented/tuned series.

A fourth aspect to such a program of prevention and optimization of music is the measurement of sound levels in various locations in the performance pit in order to ascertain the locations of intense music sound energy.

As stated in the introduction, many performance pits for musicians are unnecessarily loud, and with some manipulation, levels can be reduced.

(Place short curriculum vitae here)

References

Abel, S. M., Alberti, P. A., Haythornwaite, C., & Riko, K. (1982). Speech intelligibility in noise with and without ear protectors. In P. W. Alberti (Ed.), *Personal hearing protection in industry.* (pp. 371–386). New York: Raven Press.

Alberti, P. W. (Ed.). (1982). *Personal hearing protection in industry.* New York: Raven Press.

Ando, Y., & Gottlob, D. (1979). Effects of early multiple reflections on subjective preference judgments of music sound fields. *Journal of the Acoustical Society of America, 65,* 524–527.

Attias, J., Furst, M., Furman, V., Reshef (Haran), I., Horowitz, G., & Bresloff, I. (1995). Noise-induced otoacoustic emission loss with or without hearing loss. *Ear and Hearing, 16*(6), 612–618.

Axelsson, A., & Lindgren, F. (1978a). Temporary threshold shifts after exposure to pop music. *Scandinavian Audiology, 7,* 127–135.

Axelsson, A., & Lindgren, F. (1978b). Hearing in pop musicians. *Acta Otolaryngologica, 85,* 225–231.

Axelsson, A., & Lindgren, F. (1981). Hearing in classical musicians. *Acta Otolaryngologica* (Suppl. 377); 3–74.

Axelsson, A., Eliasson, A., & Israelsson, B. (1995). Hearing in pop/rock musicians: A follow-up study. *Ear and Hearing, 16*(3), 245–253.

Ayers, R. D. (1995). Two complex effective lengths for musical wind instruments. *Journal of the Acoustical Society of America, 98*(1), 81–87.

Bachem, A. (1955). Absolute pitch. *Journal of the Acoustical Society of America, 27,* 1180–1185.

Backus, J. (1977). *The acoustical foundations of music* (2nd ed.). New York: W.W. Norton & Company.

Barone, J. A., Peters, J. M., Garabrant, D. H., Bernstein, L., & Krebsbach, R. (1987). Smoking as a risk factor in noise-induced hearing loss. *Journal of Occupational Medicine, 29,* 741–745.

Barron, M., & Marshall, A. H. (1981). Spatial impression due to early lateral reflections in concert halls: The derivation of a physical measure. *Journal of Sound and Vibration, 77,* 211–232.

Barrs, D., Althoff, L., Krueger, W., & Olsson, J. (1994). Work-related, noise-induced hearing loss: Evaluation including evoked potential audiometry. *Otolaryngology-Head and Neck Surgery, 110*(2), 177–184.

Baughn, W. L. (1973). Relation between daily noise exposure and hearing loss as based on the evaluation of 6835 industrial noise exposure cases. Aerospace Medical Research Laboratory, Wright-Patterson Air Force Base, Dayton, Ohio, TR AMRL-TR-73-53 (AD 767 204).

Behar, A., & Desormeaux, J. (1994). NRR, ABC OR. . . . *Canadian Acoustics, 22*(1), 27–30.

Benade, A. H. (1973). The physics of brasses. *Scientific American, 229*(1), 24–35.

Benade, A. H. (1990). *Fundamentals of musical acoustics.* New York: Dover Publications, Inc.

Beranek, L. L. (1962). *Music, acoustics, and architecture.* New York: Wiley Press.

Beranek, L. L. (1986). *Acoustics*. New York: American Institute of Physics.

Beranek, L. L. (1992). Concert hall acoustics-1992. *Journal of the Acoustical Society of America, 92*(1), 1–40.

Berger, E. H. (1986). Methods of measuring the attenuation of hearing protection devices. *Journal of the Acoustical Society of America, 79*(6), 1655–1687.

Berger, E. H. (1987). Can hearing aids provide hearing protection? *E·A·R·LOG 18*. Indianapolis, IN: Cabot Safety Corporation.

Berger, E. H. (1988). Tips for fitting hearing protectors. *E·A·R·LOG·19·*. Indianapolis, IN: Cabot Safety Corporation.

Berger, E. H., & Kerivan, J. E. (1983). Influence of physiological noise and the occlusion effect on the measurement of real-ear attenuation at threshold. *Journal of the Acoustical Society of America, 74*(1), 81–94.

Berger, E. H., Royster, L. H., & Thomas, W. G. (1978). Presumed noise-induced permanent threshold shift resulting from exposure to an A-weighted Leq of 89 dB. *Journal of the Acoustical Society of America, 64*(1), 192–197.

Berlin, C. I. (1994). When outer hair cells fail, use correct circuitry to simulate their function. *Hearing Journal, 47*(4), 43.

Bies, D. A. (1994). An alternative model for combining noise and age-induced hearing loss. *Journal of the Acoustical Society of America, 95*(1), 563–565.

Bies, D. A., & Hansen, C. H. (1990). An alternative mathematical description of the relationship between noise exposure and hearing loss. *Journal of the Acoustical Society of America, 88*(6), 2743–2754.

Bohne, B. A. (1976). Safe level for noise exposure? *Annals of Otology, Rhinology, and Laryngology, 85*(1), 711–724.

Borg, E., & Counter, S. A. (1989). The middle-ear muscles. *Scientific American, 260*(8), 74–80

Borg, E., Counter, S. A., & Rosler, G. (1984). Theories of the middle-ear muscle function. In S. Silman (Ed.), *The acoustic reflex: Basic principles and clinical applications*. New York: Academic Press.

Borg, E., Nilsson, R., & Engström, B. (1983). Effect of the acoustic reflex on inner ear damage induced by industrial noise. *Acta Otolaryngologica (Stockh), 96*, 361–369.

Botsford, J. H. (1973). How to estimate dBA reduction of ear protectors. *Journal of Sound and Vibration, 6*, 32–33.

Bradley, J. S. (1990). The evolution of newer auditorium acoustics measures. *Canadian Acoustics, 18*(4), 13–23.

Bradley, J. S. (1991). Comparison of a multi-purpose hall with three well-known concert halls. *Canadian Acoustics, 19*(2), 3–10.

Caiazzo, A., & Tonndorf, J. (1977). Ear canal resonance and temporary threshold shift. *Journal of the Acoustical Society of America, 61*, 578.

Camp, J. E., & Horstman, S. W. (1992). Musician sound exposure during performance of Wagner's Ring Cycle. *Medical Problems of Performing Artists, 7*(2), 37–39.

Campbell, M., & Greated, C. (1987). *The musician's guide to acoustics*. London: J.M. Dent.

Campo, P., Subramaniam, M., & Henderson, D. (1991). Effect of "conditioning" exposures on hearing loss from traumatic exposure. *Hearing Research, 55*, 195–200.

Carlin, M. F., & McCrosky, R. L. (1980). Is the eye color a predictor of noise induced hearing loss? *Ear and Hearing, 1*(3), 191–196.

Carter, N. L. (1980). Eye color and susceptibility to noise induced permanent threshold shift. *Audiology, 19*, 86–93.

Chasin, M. (1989a). *The use of the Valsalva maneuver in some musicians to protect hearing.* Technical paper presented at the Ontario Association for Speech-Language Pathologists and Audiologists (OSLA), Toronto, Canada.

Chasin, M. (1989b). Current issues in probe tube microphone measurement. *Journal of Speech Pathology and Audiology, 13*(2), 3–11.

Chasin, M. (1994). The acoustic advantanges of CIC hearing aids. *Hearing Journal, 47*(11), 13–17.

Chasin, M. (1995a). [Spectral assessment of a Japanese drum band]. Unpublished data.

Chasin, M. (1995b). [TTS differences in Broadway-like shows]. Unpublished data.

Chasin, M., & Chong, J. (1991). In situ hearing protection program for musicians. *Hearing Instruments, 42*(12), 26–28.

Chasin, M., & Chong, J. (1992). A clinically efficient hearing protection program for musicians. *Medical Problems of Performing Artists, 7*(2), 40–43.

Chasin, M., & Chong, J. (1994). Musicians and the prevention of hearing loss. *Journal of Speech-Language Pathology and Audiology, 18*(3), 171–176.

Chasin, M., & Chong, J. (1995). Four environmental techniques to reduce the effect of music exposure on hearing. *Medical Problems of Performing Artists, 10*(2), 66–69.

Chong, J., Zaza, C., & Smith, F. C. (1991). Design and implementation of a performing artists' health program in Canada. *Medical Problems of Performing Artists, 6*(3), 8–10.

Chung, D. Y., Wilson, G. N., Gannon, P., & Mason, K. (1982). Individual susceptibility to noise. In R. P. Hamernik, D. Henderson, & R. Salvi (Eds.), *New perspectives in noise-induced hearing loss* (pp. 511–519). New York: Raven Press.

Clark, W. (1991a). Recent studies of temporary threshold shift (TTS) and permanent threshold shift (PTS) in animals. *Journal of the Acoustical Society of America, 90*(1), 155–163.

Clark, W. (1991b). Noise exposure from leisure activities: A review. *Journal of the Acoustical Society of America, 90*(1), 175–181.

Coles, R. R. A. (1987). Tinnitus and its management," In S. D. G. Stephens, & A. G. Kerr, (Eds.), *Scott Brown's Otolaryngology: Audiology*, vol. 2, (5th ed., pp. 368–414). London: Butterworth.

Cooper, J. C. (1994). Health and nutrition examination survey of 1971–75: Part I. Ear and race effects in hearing. *Journal of the American Academy of Audiology, 5*(1), 30–36.

Crow, S., Guild, S., & Polvogot, L. (1934). Observation on pathology of high-tone deafness. *Johns Hopkins Medical Journal, 54*, 315–318.

Davis, H., Morgan, C. T., Hawkins, J. T., Galambos, R., & Smith, F. W. (1950). Temporary deafness following exposure to loud tones and noise. *Acta Otolaryngologica, 88*(Suppl. 195), 1–57.

Dengerink, H. A., Lindgren, F., Axelsson, A., & Dengerink, J. E. (1987). The effects of smoking and physical exercise on temporary threshold shifts. *Scandinavian Audiology, 16*, 131–136.

Dengerink, H. A., Trueblood, G. W., & Dengerink, J. E. (1984). The effects of smoking and environmental temperature on temporary threshold shifts. *Audiology, 23,* 401–410.

Dey, F. L. (1970). Auditory fatigue and predicted permanent hearing defects from rock-and-roll music. *The New England Journal of Medicine, 282*(9), 467–470.

Embleton, T. (1995). Upper limits on noise in the workplace. Report by the International Institute of Noise Control Engineering Working Party. *Canadian Acoustics, 23*(2), 11–20.

Environmental Protection Agency. (1973). Public health and welfare criteria for noise. EPA Rep. No. 550/9-73-002.

Fletcher, H. & Munson, W. A. (1933). Loudness, its definition, measurement and calculation. *Journal of the Acoustical Society of America, 5*(1), 82–108.

Fletcher, N., & Rossing, T. (1991). *The physics of musical instruments.* New York: Springer-Verlag.

Flottorp, G. (1973). Music- A noise hazard? *Acta Otolaryngologica* (Stockh), *75,* 345–347.

Gastmeier, B., Pernu, D., & Chasin, M. (1994). *Occupational noise exposure in the high school music practice room.* Technical paper presented at the 1994 Congress of the Canadian Acoustical Association, Ottawa, Canada.

Gauthier, E., & Burak, M. (1983). Towards a high fidelity hearing aid: The folded horn. *Hearing Aid Journal, 36*(10), 37–39.

Guinan, J. J. (1986). Effect of efferent neural activity on cochlear mechanics. In G. Cianfrone & F. Grandori (Eds.), *Cochlear mechanics and otoacoustic emissions* (pp. 53–62). *Scandinavian Audiology,* Suppl. 25.

Hall, J. W., & Santucci, M. (1995). Protecting the professional ear: Conservation strategies and devices. *Hearing Journal, 48*(3), 37–45.

Hart, C. W., Geltman, C. L., Schupbach, J., & Santucci, M. (1987). The musician and occupational sound hazards. *Medical Problems of Performing Artists,* 2(3), 22–25.

Hawkins, J. E. (1971). The role of vasoconstriction in noise-induced hearing loss. *Annals of Otology, Rhinology, and Laryngology, 80,* 903–913.

Hazell, J., Jastreboff, P. J., Meerton, L. E., & Conway, M. J. (1993).Electrical tinnitus suppression: Frequency dependence of effects. *Audiology, 32,* 68–77.

Henderson, D., Hamernik, R. P., & Sitler, R. W. (1974). Audiometric and histological correlates of exposure to 1-ms noise impulses in the chinchilla. *Journal of the Acoustical Society of America, 56*(3), 1210–1221.

Henderson, D., Subramaniam, M., & Boettcher, F. A. (1993). Individual susceptibility to noise-induced hearing loss: An old topic revisited. *Ear and Hearing, 14*(3), 152–168.

Henselman, L. W., Henderson, D., Shadoan, J., Subramaniam, M., Saunders, S., & Ohlin, D. (1995). Effects of noise exposure, race, and years of service on hearing in U.S. Army soldiers. *Ear and Hearing, 16*(4), 382–391.

Hétu, R., & Fortin, M. (1995). Potential risk of hearing damage associated with exposure to highly amplified music. *Journal of the American Academy of Audiology, 6*(5), 378–387.

Hétu, R., Phaneuf, R., & Marien, C. (1987). Non-acoustic environmental factor influences on occupational hearing impairment: A preliminary discussion paper. *Canadian Acoustics, 15*(1), 17–31.

Hétu, R., Tran Quoc, H., & Tougas, Y. (1992). Can an inactivated hearing aid act as a hearing protector? *Canadian Acoustics, 20*(3), 35–36.

Hidaka, T., Beranek, L. L., & Okano, T. (1995). Interaural cross-correlation, lateral fraction, and low- and high-frequency sound levels as measures of acoustical quality in concert halls. *Journal of the Acoustical Society of America, 98*(2), 988–1007.

Hilding, A. C. (1953). Studies on otic labyrinth: Anatomic explanation for hearing dip at 4096 Hz characteristic of acoustic trauma and presbycusis. *Annals of Otology, Rhinology, and Laryngology, 62*, 950.

Hunt, F. V. (1982). *Electroacoustics: The analysis of transduction, and its historical background*. New York: American Institute of Physics.

International Organization for Standardization. (1990). *Acoustics—determination of occupational noise exposure and estimation of noise-induced hearing impairment* (2nd ed). International Standard ISO 1999.

Ismail, A. H., Corrigan, D. L., MacLeod, D. F., Anderson, V. L., Kasten, R. N., & Elliot, P. W. (1973). Biophysiological and audiological variables in adults. *Archives of Otolaryngology, 97*, 447–451.

Jansson, E., & Karlsson, K. (1983). Sound level recorded within a symphony orchestra and risk criteria for hearing loss. *Scandinavian Audiology, 12*(3), 215–221.

Jastreboff, P. J., & Hazell, J. (1993). A neurophysiological approach to tinnitus: Clinical implications. *British Journal of Audiology, 27*, 7–17.

Jerger, J., & Jerger, S. (1970). Temporary threshold shift in rock-and-roll musicians. *Journal of Speech and Hearing Research, 13*, 221–224.

Johnson, D. L. (1973). Prediction of NIPTS due to continuous noise exposure. Aerospace Medical Research Laboratory Report Number, AMRL-TR-73-91, Wright-Patterson Air Force Base, Dayton, Ohio.

Johnson, D. L. (1991). Field studies: Industrial exposures. *Journal of the Acoustical Society of America, 90*(1), 170–174.

Johnson, D. L., & Nixon, C. W. (1974). Simplified methods for estimating hearing protector performance. *Journal of Sound and Vibration, 7*, 20–27.

Johnson, D. W., Sherman, R. E., Aldridge, J., & Lorraine, A. (1985). Effects of instrument type and orchestral position on hearing sensitivity for 0.25 to 20 kHz in the orchestral musician. *Scandinavian Audiology, 14*, 215–221.

Johnson, R. M., Brummet, R., & Schleuning, A. (1993). Use of Aprazolam for relief of tinnitus. *Archives of Otolaryngology—Head and Neck Surgery, 119*, 842–845.

Karlsson, K., Lundquist, P. G., & Olaussen, T. (1983). The hearing of symphony orchestra musicians. *Scandinavian Audiology, 12*(3), 257–264.

Killion, M. C. (1993). The parvum bonum, plus melius fallacy in earplug selection. In L. Beilin, & G. R. Jensen (Eds.), Recent developments in hearing instrument technology (15th Danavox Symposium) (pp. 415–433). Scanticon, Kolding, Denmark: The Danavox Jubilee Foundation.

Killion, M. C., DeVilbiss, E., & Stewart, J. (1988). An earplug with uniform 15-dB attenuation. *Hearing Journal, 41*(5), 14–16.

Killion, M. C., Stewart, J. K., Falco, R., & Berger, E. H. (1992). Improved audibility earplug. U.S. Patent 5,113,967.

Knox, A. W. (1993). Tinnitus: A review of the literature. *Spectrum* (The National Hearing Conservation Association Newsletter), *10*(1), 1–9.

Kryter, K. D., Ward, W. D., Miller, J. D., & Eldredge, D. H. (1966). Hazardous exposures to intermittent and steady-state noise. *Journal of the Acoustical Society of America, 39*, 451–464.

Langendorf, F. G. (1992). Absolute pitch: Review and speculations. *Medical Problems of Performing Artists, 7*(1), 6–13.

Lawrence, M., Gonzales, G., & Hawkins, J. E. (1967). Some physiological factors in noise induced hearing loss. *American Industrial Hygiene Journal, 28*, 425–428.

Lebo, C. P., Oliphant, K. S., & Garrett, J. (1970). Acoustic trauma from rock-and-roll music. *California Medicine, 107*(11), 378–380.

Lempert, B. L., & Henderson, T. L. (1973). NIOSH survey of occupational noise and hearing: 1968 to 1972. U.S. Department of Health, Education and Welfare, National Institute for Occupational Safety and Health, TR 86.

Levine, R. A. (1994). Tinnitus. *Current Opinion in Otolaryngology & Head and Neck Surgery, 2*, 171–176.

Lim, D. J. (1986). Cochlear micromechanics in understanding otoacoustic emission. In G. Cianfrone & F. Grandori (Eds.), *Cochlear mechanics and otoacoustic emissions* (pp. 17–26). *Scandinavian Audiology* (Suppl. 25).

Lindau, M. (1978). Vowel features. *Language, 54*, 541–563.

Lindblad, A-C. (1982). Detection of nonlinear distortion of speech signals by hearing impaired listeners. TA105, Stockholm, Sweden, Karolinska Institute (KTH).

Lindblad, A-C. (1987). Influence of nonlinear distortion on speech intelligibility: Hearing impaired listeners. TA 116, Stockholm, Sweden, Karolinska Institute (KTH).

Lindgren, F., & Axelsson, A. (1983). Temporary threshold shift after exposure to noise and music of equal energy. *Ear and Hearing, 4*(4), 197–201.

Lonsbury-Martin, B. L., Harris, F. P., Hawkins, M. D., Stagner, B. B., & Martin, G. K. (1990). Distortion product emissions in humans II: Relations to acoustic immittance and stimulus frequency and spontaneous otoacoustic emissions in normally hearing subjects. *Annals of Otology, Rhinology, and Laryngology, 147* (Suppl. 99), 15–28.

Lonsbury-Martin, B. L., & Martin, G. K. (1990). The clinical utility of distortion product otoacoustic emissions. *Ear and Hearing, 11*, 44–154.

Lonsbury-Martin, B. L., McCoy, M. J., Whitehead, M. L., & Martin, G.(1993). Clinical testing of distortion-product otoacoustic emissions. *Ear and Hearing, 14*(1), 11–22.

Macrae, J. H. (1991). Presbycusis and noise-induced permanent threshold shift. *Journal of the Acoustical Society of America, 90*(5), 2513–2516.

Mahoney, C. F. O., & Kemp, D. (1995). Distortion product otoacoustic emission delay measurements in human ears. *Journal of the Acoustical Society of America, 97*(6), 3721–3735.

Makrinenko, L. (1994). *Acoustics of auditoriums in public buildings*. Woodbury, New York: Acoustical Society of America.

Marshall, A. H. (1967). A note on the importance of room cross-section in concert halls. *Journal of Sound and Vibration, 5*, 100–112.

Marshall, A. H. (1968). Acoustical determinents for the architectural design of concert halls. *Archives of Scientific Review*, (Australia), *11*, 81–87.

Martin, A. (1976). The equal energy concept applied to impulse noise. In D. Henderson, R. P. Hamernik, D. S. Dosanjh, & J. H. Mills (Eds.), *Effects of noise on hearing* (pp. 421–453). New York: Raven Press.

McBride, D., Gill, F., Proops, D., Harrington, M., Gardiner, K., & Attwell, C. (1992). Noise and the classical musician. *British Medical Journal, 305,* 1561–1563.

Melnick, W. (1991). Human temporary threshold shift (TTS) and damage risk. *Journal of the Acoustical Society of America, 90*(1), 147–154.

Miller, J. D., Watson, C. S., & Covell, W. P. (1963). Deafening effects of noise on the cat. *Acta Otolaryngologica,* Suppl. *176,* 1–91.

Mills, J. H., Gilbert, R. M., & Adkins, W. Y. (1979). Temporary threshold shifts in humans exposed to octave bands of noise for 16 to 24 hours. *Journal of the Acoustical Society of America, 65*(5), 1238–1248.

Mills, J. H., Osguthorpe, J. D., Burdick, C. K., Patterson, J. H., & Mozo, B.(1983). Temporary threshold shifts produced by exposure to low-frequency noises. *Journal of the Acoustical Society of America, 73,* 918–923.

Miyakita, T., Hellstrom, P. A., Frimansson, E., & Axelsson, A. (1992). Effect of low level acoustic stimulation on temporary threshold shift in young humans. *Hearing Research, 60,* 149–155.

Moore, B. C. J. (1986). Parallels between frequency selectivity measured psychophysically and in cochlear mechanics. In G. Cianfrone & F. Grandori (Eds.) *Cochlear mechanics and otoacoustic emissions* (pp. 139–152). *Scandinavian Audiology*(Suppl. 25).

Muchnick, C., Hildesheimer, M., & Rubinstein, M. (1980). Effects of emmotional stress on hearing. *Archives of Otology, Rhinology, and Laryngology, 228,* 295–298.

Murai, K., Tyler, R. S., Harker, L. A., & Stouffer, J. L. (1992). Review of pharmacologic treatment of tinnitus. *American Journal of Otology, 13,* 454–464.

Newby, P. (1990). *Real ear measurement for the hearing health care professional.* Dorchester, Ontario, Canada: Audioscan, Inc.

Nixon, C. W., Hille, H. K., & Kettler, L. K. (1967). Attenuation characteristics of earmuffs at low audio and infrasonic frequencies. Rep. AMRL-TR-67-27, Wright-Patterson Air Force Base, Dayton, OH.

Ontario Ministry of Labour. Safety guidelines for the live performance industry in Ontario. (1st ed.), Dec. 1993.

Pang-Ching, G. (1982). Hearing levels of secondary school band directors. *The Journal of Auditory Research, 22,* 284–288.

Parkin, P .H., Allen, W. A., Purkis, J., & Scholes, W. E. (1953). The acoustics of the Royal Festival Hall, London. *Acustica, 3,* 1–21.

Passchier-Vermeer, W. (1968). Hearing loss due to exposure to steady-state broadband noise, Rep. No. 35, The Netherlands, Institute for Public Health Engineering.

Passchier-Vermeer, W. (1971). Steady-state and fluctuating noise: Its effects on the hearing of people. In D. W. Robinson (Ed.), *Occupational hearing loss.* New York: Academic Press.

Patchett, R. (1992). The effects of inhalation of oxygen and carbon dioxide mixtures on noise-induced temporary threshold shift in humans. *Canadian Acoustics, 20*(1), 21–25.

Preves, D. A., & Pehringer, J. L. (1983). Calculating individuals NRRs in situ using subminiature probe microphones. *Hearing Instruments, 33*(3), 10–14.

Price, G. R. (1994). Occasional exposure to impulsive sounds: Significant noise exposure? Forum presented at the 19th annual National Hearing Conservation Association (NHCA) Conference, Atlanta, GA.

Price, G. R., & Kalb, J. T. (1991). Insights into hazard from intense impulses from a mathematical model of the ear. *Journal of the Acoustical Society of America, 90*(1), 219–227.

Prince, M. M., & Matonoski, G. M. (1991). Problems on ascertaining the combined effects of exposure: Results of an occupational cohort study of the joint effects of noise and smoking on hearing acuity. In L. Fechter (Ed.), *Proceedings of the IV international conference on the combined effects of environmental factors* (pp. 87–91). Baltimore: Johns Hopkins University.

Randall, R. B. (1977). *Application of B&K equipment to frequency analysis.* (2nd ed.). Nærum, Denmark: Bruel & Kjaer.

Rintelmann, W. F., & Borus, J. F. (1968). Noise-induced hearing loss and rock-and-roll music. *Archives of Otolaryngology, 88*(10), 377–385.

Robinson, D. W. (1968). The relationship between hearing loss and noise exposure. National Physical Laboratory Aero Rep. Ae32, England.

Robinson, D. W. (1971). Estimating the risk of hearing loss due to continuous noise. In D. W. Robinson (Ed.), *Occupational hearing loss.* New York: Academic Press.

Robinson, D. W. (1976). Characteristics of occupational noise-induced hearing loss. In D. Henderson, R. P. Hamernik, D. S. Dosanjh, & J. H. Mills (Eds.), *Effects of noise on hearing.* New York: Raven Press.

Robinson, D. W. (1988). Threshold of hearing as a function of age and sex for the typical unscreened population. *British Journal of Audiology, 22*(1), 5–20.

Roederer, J. G. (1995). *The physics and psychophysics of music: An introduction.* New York: Springer-Verlag.

Rogers, H. (1991). *Theoretical and practical phonetics.* Toronto, Canada: Copp Clark Pitman, Ltd.

Rosenberg, P. E. (1978). Case history: The first test. In J. Katz (Ed.), *Handbook of clinical audiology* (2nd ed.) (pp. 77–80). Baltimore: The Williams and Wilkins Company.

Rosenhall, U., Pedersen, K., & Svanborg, A. (1990). Presbycusis and noise-induced hearing loss. *Ear and Hearing, 11*(4), 257–263.

Rosowski, J. (1991). The effects of external- and middle-ear filtering on auditory threshold and noise-induced hearing loss. *Journal of the Acoustical Society of America, 90*(1), 124–135.

Royster-Doswell, J., Royster, L., & Killion, M. (1991). Sound exposures and hearing thresholds of symphony orchestra muscians. *Journal of the Acoustical Society of America, 89*(6), 2793–2803.

Sanden, A., & Axelsson, A. (1981). Comparison of cardiovascular responses in noise-resistant and noise-sensitive workers. *Acta Otolaryngology* (Stockh), *76* (Suppl. 377), 75–100.

Sataloff, R. T., & Sataloff, J. (Eds.). (1995). *Occupational hearing loss* (2nd ed.). New York: Marcel Dekker Inc.

Schroeter, J. (1986). The use of acoustical test fixtures for the measurement of hearing protector attenuation. Part I: Review of previous work and the design of an improved test fixture. *Journal of the Acoustical Society of America, 79,* 1065–1081.

Schuknecht, H., & Tonndorf, J. (1960). Acoustic trauma of the cochlea from ear surgery. *Laryngoscope, 70,* 479.

Selters, W., & Ward, W. D. (1962). Temporary threshold shift with changing duty cycles. *Journal of the Acoustical Society of America, 34,* 122–123.

Shaw, E. A. G., & Theissen, G. J. (1958). Improved cushion for ear defenders. *Journal of the Acoustical Society of America, 30,* 24–36.

Shaw, E. A. G., & Theissen, G. J. (1962). Acoustics of circumaural earphones. *Journal of the Acoustical Society of America, 34,* 1233–1243.

Sivan, L. J. & White, S. D. (1933). On minimum audible fields. *Journal of the Acoustical Society of America, 4,* 288–321.

Speaks, C., Nelson, D., & Ward, W. D. (1970). Hearing loss in rock-and-roll musicians. *Journal of Occupational and Environmental Medicine, 12*(6), 216–219.

Spoendlin, H. (1986). Receptoneural and innervation aspects of the inner ear anatomy with respect to cochlear mechanics. In G. Cianfrone & F. Grandori (Eds.), *Cochlear mechanics and otoacoustic emissions* (pp. 27–34). *Scandinavian Audiology* (Suppl. 25).

Stevens, S. S. (1961). Procedure for calculating loudness. *Journal of the Acoustical Society of America, 33,* 1577–1585.

Subramaniam, M., Henderson, D., & Spongr, V. (1991). Frequency differences in the development fo protection against NIHL by low level "toughening" exposures. *Journal of the Acoustical Society of America, 89*(4, Part 2), 1865–1874.

Swanson, S. J., Dengerink, H. A., Kondrick, P., & Miller, C. L. (1987). The influence of subjective factors on temporary threshold shifts after exposure to music and noise of equal energy. *Ear and Hearing, 8*(5), 288–291.

Taylor, W., Pearson, J., Mair, W., & Burns, W. (1965). Study of noise and hearing in jute weaving. *Journal of the Acoustical Society of America, 38,* 113–120.

Titze, I. R. (1995). *Mechanisms of vocal vibrato.* Technical paper presented at the Acoustical Society of America , 130th Meeting, St. Louis, MO.

Tonndorf, J. (1976). Relationship between the transmission characteristics of conductive system and noise-induced hearing loss. In D. Henderson, R. P. Hamernik, D. S. Dosanjh, & J. H. Mills, (Eds.), *Effects of noise on hearing* (pp. 159-178). New York: Raven Press.

Tyler, R. S., Aran, J-M., & Dauman, R. (1992, November). Recent advances in tinnitus. *American Journal of Audiology,* 36–43.

United States Department of Labor, Occupational Safety and Health Administration. (1981). Occupational noise exposure: hearing conservation amendment, Part III. *Federal Reg., 46,* 4078–4179.

Vittitow, M., Windmill, I. M., Yates, J. W., & Cunningham, D. R. (1994). Effect of simultaneous exercise and noise exposure (music) on hearing. *Journal of the American Academy of Audiology, 5*(5), 343–348.

Wallach, H., Newman, E. B., & Rosenzweig, M. R. (1949). The precedence effect in sound localization. *American Journal of Psychology, 62,* 315.

Ward, W. D. (1970). Temporary threshold shift and damage risk criteria for intermittent noise exposures. *Journal of the Acoustical Society of America, 48,* 561–574.

Ward, W. D. (1974). Noise levels are not noise exposures! Proceedings of NOIS-EXPO Conference, 170–175.

Ward, W. D. (1976). A comparison of the effects of continuous, intermittent and impulse noise. In D. Henderson, R. P. Hamernik, D. S. Dosanjh, & J. H. Mills (Eds.), *Effects of noise on hearing* (pp. 407–420). New York: Raven Press.

Ward, W. D. (1982). Summation of international symposium on hearing protection in industry. In P. A. Alberti (Ed.), *Personal hearing protection in industry* (pp. 577–592). New York: Raven Press.

Ward, W. D. (1991). The role of intermittence in PTS. *Journal of the Acoustical Society of America, 90*(1), 164–169.

Ward, W. D., Cushing, E. M., & Burns, E. M. (1976). Effective quiet and moderate TTS: Implications for noise exposure standards. *Journal of the Acoustical Society of America, 59*, 160–165.

West, P. D. B., & Evans, E. F. (1990). Early detection of hearing damage in young listeners resulting from exposure to amplified music. *British Journal of Audiology, 24*, 89–103.

Westmore, G. A., & Eversden, I. D. (1981). Noise-induced hearing loss and orchestral musicians. *Archives of Otolaryngology, 107*, 761–764.

Yassi, A., Pollock, N., Tran, N., & Cheang, M. (1993). Risks to hearing from a rock concert. *Canadian Family Physician, 39*(5), 1045–1049.

Yost, W., & Nielsen, D. (1985). *Fundamentals of hearing: An introduction* (2nd ed.). New York: Holt, Rinehart and Winston.

Zakrisson, J-E, Borg, E., Liden, G., & Nilsson, R. (1980). Stapedius reflex in industrial impact noise: Fatigability and role for temporary threshold shift (TTS). *Scandinavian Audiology* (Suppl. 12), 326–334.

Zwislocki, J. (1953). Acoustic attenuation between the ears. *Journal of the Acoustical Society of America, 25*, 752–759.

Zwislocki, J. (1957). In search of the bone-conduction threshold in a free sound field. *Journal of the Acoustical Society of America, 29*, 795–804.

Index

A

Acoustic monitoring devices, 136–137
Acoustic transformer effect, 54–56
Acoustics,
  of churches, 127–128
  of community halls, 128–129
  of performance halls, 121–127
  of rehearsal rooms, 127
  of theaters, 128
Advocacy and educational organizations, 168
Amplified instruments, sound-reducing strategies, 142–144
Attenuation characteristics, 84–87
  of hearing protectors, 111–113, 160
    assessment techniques, 96–97
Audiologist evaluation form, 162–166
Audiometric assessment, of musicians, 106–107
Auditory toughening, 37–39

B

Baffles, 122–124, 130
Baritone, 74–75
Bars, 78–79
Bass, 75–78
Bassoon, 67–71, 139–140
Boundary conditions, 63
Bournoulli principle, 54–55, 67, 69
Bowed stringed instruments, 62, 75–78
  and optimal hearing protection, 93, 94
Brass instruments, 62, 72–75
  and optimal hearing protection, 93, 94
  sound level reducing strategies, 137–139

C

Case history, in musician hearing assessment, 103–106
Cello, 75–78, 117–118, 136–137
Churches, acoustics, 121, 123, 127–128
Clarinet, 67–71, 139–140
Clouds, 122–124, 130
Cochlea. *See* Inner ear.
Committee on Hearing and Bioacoustics (CHABA), 26, 28, 31
Community halls, acoustics, 128–129
Conductive hearing losses, 14
Cymbals, 79

D

Damping, 52–53
Diplacusis, 1, 22
Distortion, 5–8, 23. *See also* Harmonic distortion.

E

Ear
  anatomy, 9
  inner ear, 14–16
  middle ear, 11–14
  outer ear, 9–11
Ear plugs. *See* Hearing protection.
Earphones, 143–144, 145
  manufacturers, 167
Efferent nerve fibres, 15–16
Electrical amplification systems, 122, 126, 129–130
Electronic-based hearing protection, 95–96
English horn, 67–71
Equal loudness contours, 1, 18–20, 23
ER-series earplugs, 87–92, 111, 115–116, 134, 139, 140, 146
  attenuation characteristics, 160
Exchange rate, 31–32

F

Fast Fourier Transforms, 2–3, 5, 110
Fluegel horn, 74–75

Flute, 71–72, 139–140
and optimal hearing protection, 93, 94
Flutter echo, 123–124
Fourier analysis, 2–3
French horn, 73–75, 137–139
Frequency, 2, 4
Fundamental frequency, 21
Fundamental tracking, 8

G

Genetic factors, and hearing loss, 39
Glockenspiel, 78–79
Gongs, 78–79
Government agencies, 152–153
Greek amphitheaters, acoustics, 121–122

H

Hair cells, 14–16
Half wavelength resonators, 48–51
and the piano, 65
Harmonic distortion, 5–8, 23
Harp, 136
Harpsichord, 65, 66–67
Health professionals, occupational health education, 155
Hearing assessment, of musicians, 103
audiometric assessment, 106–107
case history use, 103–106
case scenarios, 114–118
remedial recommendations, 111
spectral assessment of instruments, 107–111
verification of attenuation characteristics, 111–113
verification of degree of occlusion effect, 113–114
Hearing loss,
education organizations, 153
reducing strategies, 161
Hearing protection,
acoustically tuned alternatives, 87–92
attenuation assessment techniques, 96–97
attenuation characteristics, 84–87
electronic based, 95–96
ER-series earplugs, 87–92
nonpersonal methods, 99–100, 101
optimal musician protection, 92–95
single value attenuation rating schemes, 97–99
Helmholtz resonance, 3–4, 51–52, 71, 75
vocal tract, 80
High-frequency emphasis, 134
High-frequency reflectivity/impedance, 56–57
Human voice, acoustic characteristic, 79–81
Human performance prevention model, 149–152, 154

I

Impedance matching, 11
Impulse noise, 30–31
Inner ear, 14–16, 18
Insertion loss, 96, 112
Intermodulation distortion, 8–9
International Organization for Standardization, 29–30

L

Loudness, 4, 20–21
Loudness summation, 1, 20–21
Loudspeakers, placement, 142–144

M

Mechanical resonances, 51–52
Middle ear, 11–14
Musical instruments,
acoustic characteristics, 61–64
acoustic transformer effect, 54–56
brass, 72–75
flute, 70–72
percussion, 78–79
piano, 65–67
reeded woodwinds, 67–71
spectral assessment, 107–111

stringed, 75–78
Musical note-to-frequency chart, 2, 22–23, 64, 157, 158
Musicians,
education, 153–155
hearing loss reduction strategies, 148
music-induced hearing loss, 16–18
optimal hearing protection, 92–95, 159
personal role in hearing protection, 149–152

N

Noise-induced hearing loss models, 29–32
Noise Reduction Rating (NRR), 97–99
Nonpersonal hearing protection methods, 99–100, 101

O

Oboe, 67–71, 139–140
Occlusion effect, 84, 85
degree verification, 113–114
and musicians, 87
Orchestras,
average spectra, 33–35
sample proposal, 168–170
Otoacoustic emissions, 16, 20, 35, 104, 107, 108
Outer ear, 9–11

P

Percussion instruments, 62, 78–79, 116–117
sound reduction strategies, 140–142
Performance halls, acoustics, 121–127
Performing artist. *See* Musicians *or* Vocalists.
Permanent threshold shift, 26–28
auditory toughening, 37–39
exchange rates, 31–32
prediction models, 29–30, 31
Phonemic spectrum, 62–63
Phonetic spectrum, 62–63
Piano, 62, 65–67
Pitch, 4–5, 8
Plastic shields, as hearing protectors, 99–100

Q

Quarter wavelength resonators, 46–47
brass instruments, 73–75
and ear canal, 86
reeded woodwinds, 67–71
vocal tract, 80

R

Real ear attenuation at threshold, 97
of ear plugs, 112–113
Real ear measurement (REM) system, 107–110
occlusion effect measurement, 113–114
Real ear unaided response, 86
Reeded woodwinds, 62, 67–71
and optimal hearing protection, 93, 94
Rehearsal rooms, acoustics, 127
Resonance, 44–52
half wavelength resonators, 48–51
Helmholtz resonators, 51–52
mechanical resonators, 51–52
quarter wavelength resonators, 46–47
Reverberation time, 124–125, 131

S

Sabine, Wallace, 121, 124
Saxophone, 67–71
Shakers, 141
Singers. *See* Vocalists.
Single Number Rating, 97
Smoking, and hearing loss, 40–41
Sound directivity, 57–58
Sound reflection, in performance halls, 122–123
Source-Formant-Filter-Radiation model, 63–64, 72, 79

Spectral intensity, 33–35
Standing waves, 45, 53–54
Stapedius reflex, 12–14
Starting phase, 2, 4, 5
Stringed instruments, sound level reducing strategies, 134–137

T

Temporary threshold shift, 26–29
  auditory toughening, 37–39
  and musicians, 35
  subjective factors, 36–37
Theaters, acoustics, 128
Tinnitus, 21–22, 23, 26, 106, 114
Training effect, 37–39
Trombone, 73–75, 137–139
Trumpet, 73–75, 137–139
Tympani, 78–79

V

Vibrato, 54
Viola, 75–78, 134–135
Violin, 75–78, 114–116, 134–135
Vent-associated resonance, 92
Vocal strain, 144–147
Vocal tract, acoustic characteristics, 79–81
Vocalists, 144–146
  acoustic spectra, 81–82
  optimal hearing protection, 93, 95

W

Wavelength resonances, 45–52
Woodwind instruments,
  flute, 70–72
  reeded, 67–71
  sound level reducing strategies, 139–140
Wrist-arm injury, 147